COMPLEMENTARY FEEDING:
NUTRITION, CULTURE AND POLITICS

Gabrielle Palmer is a nutritionist and is the author of the book *The Politics of Breastfeeding*, also published by Pinter & Martin. A breastfeeding counsellor in the 1970s, she later went on to help establish the UK IBFAN group, Baby Milk Action. In the early 1980s she worked in Mozambique. She has written and campaigned on infant feeding issues, particularly the unethical marketing of baby foods. In the 1990s she co-directed the International Breastfeeding: Practice and Policy Course at the Institute of Child Health in London, until she went to live in China for two years.

She has worked independently for various health and development agencies, including serving as HIV and Infant Feeding Officer for UNICEF New York. She recently worked at the London School of Hygiene and Tropical Medicine where she originally studied nutrition. She is a mother and a grandmother.

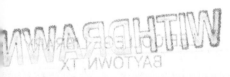

COMPLEMENTARY FEEDING: NUTRITION, CULTURE AND POLITICS

Gabrielle Palmer

pinter
&
martin

Complementary Feeding: Nutrition, Culture and Politics

Based on Gabrielle Palmer's paper *What is complementary feeding? A philosophical reflection to help a policy process* © IBFAN-GIFA, 2009

This edition first published in Great Britain by Pinter & Martin Ltd 2011

ISBN 978-1-905177-42-4

British Library Cataloguing-in-Publication Data
A catalogue record for this book is available from the British Library

Printed in Great Britain by TJ International Ltd, Padstow, Cornwall

Pinter & Martin Ltd
6 Effra Parade
London SW2 1PS

www.pinterandmartin.com

CONTENTS

PART THREE: PROCESSES FOR CHANGE

APPENDICES

INTRODUCTION

If you are looking for a strict set of instructions on how to feed your baby or toddler, put this book down immediately. However, if you are curious about the world, its children and their nutrition, buy this at once. This small book is based on a paper I wrote for the International Baby Food Action Network (IBFAN). For over thirty years this organisation has been working to halt the unethical marketing of baby foods. Its main brief has been the protection of breastfeeding and safer artificial feeding through the global implementation of the WHO/UNICEF International Code of Marketing.[1]

Many people are aware of the controversies surrounding the aggressive promotion of substitutes for breastmilk but when it comes to the food that a child eats when she needs more than milk, the whole world is in a muddle. IBFAN wanted to work out its own policy on complementary feeding so I wrote this to stimulate discussion, ideas and more investigation.

I hope that you, inquiring reader, will not take anything I have written as an absolute truth. Rather, I hope that these words will prompt you to poke into the great pot of information and misinformation that marks our age and work out for yourself what is nonsense and what is sense.

ACKNOWLEDGEMENTS

I warmly thank Adriano Cattaneo, Joanne Csete, Peter Greaves, Yasmin Hosny, Alison Jones, Lida Lhotska, Alison Linnecar, Rebecca Norton, Gill Rapley and Judith Richter, for their comments, information, suggestions and encouragement.

I warmly thank the children, parents, grandparents, photographers and colleagues for their photos. I thank UNICEF for the photos on pages 26 and 53.

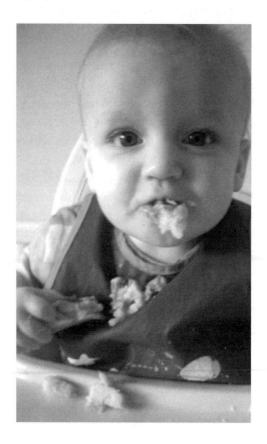

FOREWORD

"All that area was wooded. There were small farms, full of maize, millet, sorghum. The rivers were huge and clean. There was no tea. Today we see tea, tea, tea. Mother never planted tea. Tea has become slave labour."

Environmentalist and Nobel Prize winner Wangari Maathai, describing changes in the area in Kenya where she grew up (2009)[1]

Almost thirty years ago in Mozambique, I was teaching mothers of malnourished infants and young children how to improve complementary feeding.* We were in the garden of a health post under some shade trees. Two incidents haunt me to this day. The first was that a woman stood up and said: *"Thank you for this information – please could you tell us how we can get the food."* The second was that, as I was turning the flip chart of Ministry of Health teaching materials, out of the corner of my eye I saw a woman pick up a dead bird from the undergrowth, brush the dust off its feathers and pop it into her shopping basket. I should have used that opportunity to point out that small wild animals could provide some of the nutrients that the staple food of maize meal lacked.** Indecision, and fear of embarrassing her, inhibited me

---

* By complementary feeding I mean the addition of other foods to the diet of an infant or young child who is either breastfed or fed with expressed breastmilk or a breastmilk substitute. I avoid the word 'weaning' because it lacks clarity. Some interpret weaning as the addition of other foods to breastfeeding or feeding with breastmilk substitutes, while others use it to mean stopping breastfeeding. The international health agencies WHO and UNICEF also avoid this word.

** There is a risk of hand to mouth pathogenic contamination from touching a dead bird, but thorough cooking (which was the norm in that area) would render it safe for eating. Hand washing after handling the bird would be

and I let the moment go.

The important lessons that these women taught me were that, firstly, food availability is more important than knowledge and that the reverse is cruel; secondly, that millions of mothers have been able to feed their children for thousands of years without input from experts.

Having read many official documents on complementary feeding, I long to tear them into shreds and throw them out of the window. Around the world in both rich and poor regions are numerous human beings who are alive and healthy. They are the evidence that mothers (and other family members) have been able to feed their children successfully. In 2009, the press reported the world's oldest man to be 113-year-old Henry Allingham.* He was born in 1896 in a poor area of London and, during his second year, his father died of tuberculosis. Whatever his mother did can only be judged to have been the right thing.

This book does not set out to draw conclusions, make prescriptions or give practical guidance or recommendations; its purpose is to stimulate thought and debate about the subject of complementary feeding. In order to do this I will present a range of topics, facts and comment which I hope will achieve this purpose and help the necessary discussion by moving beyond the confinement of deference to the powerful, the expectations of those who hold the purse strings, political fashion and cultural inhibition.

---

desirable as infection would be through touch rather than consumption. In parts of Europe, game birds are suspended for two or three weeks to facilitate breakdown of the flesh by intrinsic bacteria. This process is favoured by gourmets for improving the flavour and texture of the meat. Game meat is customarily well cooked.

* At 113 years old, Henry Allingham was proclaimed the oldest man in the world by Guinness World Records. He died on the 18th July 2009.

PART ONE
THE BIG PICTURE

PART ONE

I

ENTITLEMENT TO FOOD

In his seminal book *Poverty and Famines,* Nobel Prize winning economist Amartya Sen introduced his theory of entitlement. This simple and compelling concept shows that people suffer hunger and die, not from lack of food, but from lack of entitlement to food. For example during the 19th century famines in Ireland, grain was exported to England. The Irish died because they depended on potatoes and the crop failed when blight disease struck. The Irish had no entitlement to the grain crops which they grew as land rent for the English landowners.[1]

Today, a traveller from a rich country might trek in a remote, drought-ridden area of the world. The traveller carries credit cards, cash and mobile phone (to call family, colleagues or bank) so that, should he lose his food supplies, he has entitlement to food when he reaches a store or eating place. An East African pastoralist family whose animals have died in a drought and who trek to seek help have no money or credit to buy food. They have no entitlement. During famines, you do not see TV journalists, politicians or aid workers fainting with hunger. Their children are unlikely to become undernourished, even if their parents are working in the famine zone, because they have entitlement to food.

This situation is echoed in conditions of entrenched poverty where a mother may have to choose between paying an older child's school fees or buying something nutritious for her toddler. In many societies women are obliged by custom to give the best food to the male family members. Children are inadequately fed for many reasons, but families' lack of entitlement through poverty, which impedes access to sufficient food of quality to meet nutritional needs, is a significant cause. The political failure to address the issue of the right to food[2] affects young children more than any other group.

Entitlement to food is also impeded by misinformation about infant and young child feeding. This is widespread, through both cultural attitudes and marketing. The former may endorse entrenched beliefs, taboos and restrictions which deprive children of a diverse and nutrient-dense diet; the latter may do the same through the marketing of unsuitable or unnecessary foods. The two often interact and modern marketing methods may both exploit and shape misguided cultural attitudes.

One harmful effect of marketing is that inexpensive local foods may be disregarded because persuasive promotional tactics convince families that, for example, a pureed banana in a jar is nutritionally superior to one in the local market. This bleeds a family's food budget, leading to restricted access to foods. Other children and a mother herself may be deprived because scarce cash is squandered on the costly industrially processed product. This confidence trick obliterates a family's entitlement to sufficient, suitable foods.

2

ENTITLEMENT TO WATER

The world seems to be in a flurry of activity to provide technical solutions to human problems while often sidestepping the causes of these problems. Some technical solutions may result in unforeseen consequences. One example could be the inappropriate promotion of Ready-to-Use Therapeutic Foods (RUTFs).* These products were invented by scientists to save the lives of severely malnourished children in emergencies. They are effective and useful products, designed to be used in health facilities under the supervision of health professionals. The manufacturers of RUTFs are now producing Ready-to-Use Supplemental Foods (RUSFs) and commercial marketing is being discussed.[1]

This pattern of market expansion echoes the history of infant formula use. Invented over a century ago, these artificial milks were intended to save the lives of a minority of infants in extreme circumstances and to be used only under the supervision of a health professional. The lure of high profits led to intensive mass marketing and widespread misuse. Health professionals and health systems got caught up in this marketing. This situation

---

* *"The first form of RUTF was invented in the late 1990s. Products qualifying to be called RUTF are energy-dense mineral- and vitamin-enriched foods equivalent in formulation to Formula 100 (F100), which is recommended by WHO for the treatment of malnutrition in in-patient settings. However, recent studies have shown that RUTF promotes faster recovery from severe acute malnutrition than standard F100. It has little available water (low water activity), which means that it is microbiologically safe, will keep for several months in simple packaging and can be made easily using low-tech production methods. RUTF is eaten uncooked, and is an ideal vehicle to deliver many micronutrients that might otherwise be broken down by cooking. RUTF is useful to treat severe malnutrition without complications in communities with limited access to appropriate local diets for nutritional rehabilitation."* Taken from http://whqlibdoc.who.int/publications/2009/9789241597494_eng.pdf

persists today, undermining breastfeeding and the responsible use of breastmilk substitutes when necessary. This subverts infant and child nutrition and women's health across the world.[2]

One article about the use of RUTFs addresses the fact that 3.5 million children die each year from undernutrition. This same text extols the links between commercial entities and health agencies, known as public-private partnerships, and states that "*Preparation of Ready-to-Use Therapeutic Foods (RUTFs) does not require water. This means that bacteria cannot grow in them and they can be used safely in people's homes.*"[3] The lower water content of both RUTFs and RUSFs may reduce the risk of bacterial contamination within the product itself but this does not cancel out the child's need for water. Indeed the child is supposed to drink plenty of clean, fresh water alongside the consumption of these foods. How do they get this water?

A reliable water supply is a key component of good complementary feeding. There are two reasons for this. The first is that a child needs water to drink. A child who is breastfeeding can get all the water she needs from her mother's milk, which is one of the many reasons that continued breastfeeding beyond two years is so important in areas of water scarcity. But many children stop breastfeeding too soon and they must drink water when their diet is comprised of solid foods.

Artificial milks such as infant formula are almost impossible to use in the areas where most malnutrition and undernutrition occurs. It is too risky to attempt artificial feeding in conditions of extreme poverty but even in rich societies, mixing powdered milk to the correct proportion of water to nutrients can be a tricky business. In the 20th century artificially fed babies in rich countries suffered and died from dehydration because their infant formula feeds contained too high a solute load. In other words, there were too many waste nutrients for a child's immature kidneys to process and these infants became dangerously dehydrated.[4] Mothers and carers were sometimes blamed for mixing too little water with the milk powder. Under pressure from doctors dealing with the ill effects, the manufacturers eventually changed the recipe of the infant formulas.

Getting the balance of water to nutrients just right is not always easy. In many traditional societies, infants and young children are given sloppy gruels made up of the local starchy staple food.* These gruels are too dilute and lack sufficient energy, protein and micronutrients. In contrast RUTFs and RUSFs are nutrient dense and low in water. RUTFs and RUSFs are made in the form of pastes, compressed bars and biscuits. Their typical ingredients are milk powder, high-quality vegetable oil, peanut paste, sugar and added nutrients. These products may actually increase a child's need for safe water to drink. Breastmilk adjusts its water content according to the surrounding climate. Once a child has stopped breastfeeding someone has to ensure the availability of alternative fluids. A young child will feel thirst when he needs to drink, but not all carers can discern between hunger and thirst. The majority of the world's population has no access to clean, safe water and boiling every drop to drink uses up scarce and expensive fuel. If an RUTF or RUSF is being used in the home, then extra fuel must be used to boil the extra water the child needs and someone must ensure that the child drinks it.

The second reason for the importance of water is that consistent supplies are essential for hygienic food preparation. Hand washing after defecation or cleaning a child's bottom, and regular bathing, are all essential to reduce the common infections, especially gastrointestinal diseases, which exacerbate undernutrition and malnutrition.

A key difference in the experience of daily life between industrialised and developing countries is water provision. Public provision of water and sanitation systems transformed the lives of families in industrialised nations during the 20th century and contributed to declines in disease long before other modern healthcare strategies, such as immunisation, were developed.

---

* These might be grain based such as rice, maize, sorghum, wheat, root based such as cassava, yams, potato or starch fruit such as plantain, banana or bread fruit.

In the 21st century a poor mother in North America, Europe or other developed regions can take a water tap in her home for granted. In rural Africa less than 6% of the population has even a communal pump or tap.[5] The Convention on the Rights of the Child claims as a right *"the provision of adequate nutritious foods and clean drinking water".*[6] Most children cannot claim this right because such water provision does not exist.

The Global Strategy for Infant and Young Child Feeding mentions water only in statements referring to *"exceptionally difficult circumstances".*[7] However, lack of access to water is not exceptional but normal for over a billion people. A target of Goal 7 of the Millennium Development Goals is to halve the proportion of people without sustainable access to safe drinking water and basic sanitation by 2015.[8] This implies acceptance of the fact that by 2015 around 500 million people will not have this access.

Water quantity and access has a greater effect on health than safe drinking water. Placing a water tap close to a home nearly doubles the chances that a mother will clean her hands after contact with her child's faeces. For drinking water, home disinfection is feasible through boiling, or through exposing water in plastic containers to sunlight, but to use water effectively for hygiene you need to be sure of a regular, adequate supply.* The definition of 'improved access' to water used for the Millennium Development Goals is a water source less than half a mile (0.8km) away. So even 'good' water access can take an hour a day of women's time. Many spend far longer – time they might spend 'actively' feeding their children (as they are urged to do).[9]

However scientifically sophisticated a manufactured foodstuff might be it cannot be anything but a stopgap measure when the environment which causes the malnutrition and undernutrition in the first place is not reformed. Even with adequate foods, whether home made or commercially manufactured, safe

---

* Average use by an individual in an industrialised country is about 200 litres a day (toilet flushing uses 15 to 26 litres). Average use by an individual in a poor country is 10 litres per day.

complementary feeding cannot be achieved if hand washing and other aspects of food hygiene are constrained through inadequate water provision.

3

MEDICALISING UNDERNUTRITION
AND POVERTY

The article about public-private partnerships and RUTFs mentioned on page 16 continues: "*Also health staff can prescribe Ready-to-Use Therapeutic Foods, decreasing the pressure on in-patient health facilities.*"[1] Several child health agencies and centres of academic research share this approach to child feeding. This reflects the sad state of affairs in the 21st century, where undernutrition in poor countries has come to be viewed as a matter of medical prescription through healthcare systems rather than an issue of food security. Furthermore, this approach disregards the fact that the families of the most vulnerable children have inadequate access to healthcare facilities. Families might live too far from a clinic. They might be deterred by costs, because even if there are no direct charges for a consultation, transport, medicines and food while they are absent from home may be beyond a family's income. In many regions clinics are scarce in number. Those that exist may be understaffed, ill-equipped and underresourced. It is usually the regions with the worst health systems that suffer the most malnutrition.

Governments, United Nations agencies and non-governmental organisations sometimes unwittingly convey in their messages an acceptance that poverty is inevitable. The proportional reduction targets of the Millennium Development Goals do not even dare present the vision of poverty eradication. This does not mean that the people who devised these goals lacked ideals but that they had to be realistic. They knew that many governments would be unwilling or unable to achieve these basic targets.

Yes, the majority of human beings are poor but they need

not be.* Certainly it would be possible for access to water and nutritious food for all to be defined as a priority before any other economic measure of prosperity. The current reality of the state of human society shames us all because we have the means to change it.

The use of a ready-made food designed for the clinical rehabilitation of severe malnutrition (RUTF) should not become the daily diet of the masses just because political leaders and public authorities neglect their basic duty to provide water, support locally sustainable food systems and communicate practical nutrition information. Another danger of the promotion and provision of such foods is that their use, beyond therapeutic feeding in emergencies, crushes a central value of human relationships and cultures: that of a family's skill to feed itself and include its youngest members in food sharing.

In a 2010 article, economist Jeffery Sachs, nutritionist Jessica Fanzo and paediatrician Sonia Sachs expressed concern about the use of RUTFs beyond their very specialised use. Amongst other disadvantages, they addressed the economic realities: *". . . it would in any event be an impossibly high cost for a 'solution' to hunger based on food aid! Suppose that the billion hungry people in the world were put on a permanent Plumpy'Nut[**2] diet (a totally misguided idea) at a cost of $30 per month, or $360 per year. The result would be a direct cost of some $360 billion per year, an absurdly high cost compared to the real solutions of improved local agriculture, improved household dietary practices, and expanded access of the poor to basic healthcare."* [3]

---

*   According to the NGO Christian Aid, ending poverty is a *"big task but no bigger than ending slavery or putting man on the moon"*. The UN Secretary General has categorically stated that it can happen. See christianaid.org.uk

**   Plumpy'Nut is the brand name of a widely distributed RUTF.

4

FAIR DISTRIBUTION

In the early 20th century, a British politician was advising a crowd of poor workers that a family could make a nourishing meal out of a cod's head. A man in the crowd shouted out: *"Who ate the cod?"* This situation is now echoed globally. Two billion people are hungry and one billion eat far too much. Countries with unacceptable levels of childhood undernutrition export food to rich countries. It takes 3,000 litres of water to produce a kilo of rice and 16,000 litres to produce a kilo of beef. The manufacture of one hamburger uses up 11,000 litres of water.[1]

Who is eating the beef? News reports from the UN and analysts in India, Washington and London estimate that 30 million hectares of farmland is being 'acquired' from the world's poor to grow food for rich countries.[2] The food systems and eating practices of the industrialised nations do indeed take food *"out of the mouths of babes and sucklings"*.*

The Chief Scientific Advisor to the British Government, Sir John Beddington, calls for 'food literacy' and states that there must be a radical redesign of the global food system because the current system is not viable. Agriculture uses 70% of the world's fresh water and contributes to 10% to 12% of greenhouse gases. Land conversion, animal grazing and nitrogenous fertilisers are the main culprits. Half of the 11.5 billion hectares of land used for agriculture is degraded. In poor countries 30% of food is lost before harvest, in rich countries 30% is wasted by the consumer.[3]

Such products as RUTFs and RUSFs are part of this food system. Designed to treat severe malnutrition, they are useful

---

* *The Bible*: Psalm 8, verse 2.

tools among a range of life-saving strategies, but the promotion of their use for everyday life must be challenged. To address nutrition problems through the mass provision of pills and products is to treat humans like farm animals. Most humans are poor and by 2050, eight out of nine billion will live in 'developing' countries. If such emergency provision is 'brought up to scale' it will lead to a world where most children are fed with an industrialised mass-produced food in the same way that battery chickens are fed with pellets. Someone will be profiting from this degradation. We have to meet the root causes head on.

This quotation from the great writer Leo Tolstoy* in 1886 describes the stance of the powerful and mimics the current state of such attitudes to complementary feeding:

"I sit on a man's back, choking him and making him carry me, and yet assure myself and others that I am very sorry for him and wish to ease his lot by all possible means . . . except by getting off his back."[4]

---

*   The Russian Leo Tolstoy (1828-1910) is famous for major novels such as *War and Peace* and *Anna Karenina*.

5

WHAT IS COMPLEMENTARY FEEDING?

Older babies and young children need foods other than breastmilk for two reasons: firstly for nutrition to grow and develop healthily; secondly to accustom them to the eating habits of the family and community. These two goals do not always harmonise. Spoon-feeding a baby a nutritionally programmed pre-packaged food while she sits in her high chair separately from the family meal excludes her from the social and emotional interactions of that meal. This is commonplace in modern, industrialised society and deprives the baby of the various taste, texture and interactive experiences of sharing the family's food. However, in some societies, the shared family meal may not deliver appropriate nutrients to the young child and she may miss out nutritionally if parents and caregivers are unaware of the importance of active feeding* and do not know which foods are the most appropriate.

Food distribution within the family does not always favour children, even in richer societies. Almost seventy years ago, the British government ran an advertising campaign called *'Don't let Dad get all the meat'* (see Appendix III). Today, even well-educated families may deprive their children of a diverse diet because marketing and misinformation lead them to believe that children need special foods in jars and packets. How infants and young children are introduced to foods is crucial for child survival and lifelong health. The process also has emotional and psychological effects and is part of acculturation,** which is one of several learning processes which help a child to become part of his group, whether family or community.

---

*   By 'active feeding' I do not mean forcing a child to eat food, but offering the best bits of the family meal and encouraging a child to feed herself.
**   Acculturation is the process of assimilation of the cultural traits of a group.

Dietary practices influence not only the development of the older baby and young child but also lifelong eating practices. In the poor world many children who are beautifully breastfed beyond two years become malnourished or die for lack of nutritious complementary foods. In the rich world many children's early feeding experiences programme them for lifelong harmful eating practices. Taste preferences are formed in early life and the content and manner of feeding may establish lifelong cravings for overly sweet, salty or energy-dense/nutrient-poor foods and drinks. Family and health worker pressures to eat too much may override innate appetite control and lead to overweight and obesity. Anorexia nervosa, bulimia and other eating disorders might even have their origins in early childhood.

There is also a confusing overlap between what are termed 'complementary foods' and what are in reality breastmilk substitutes. Even after six months, many foods do not 'complement' (ie complete) breastfeeding, but replace it, when ideally it should continue to provide the principal food. For example a baby may be fed a starchy staple, mashed fruits, juices, soups and gruels. These fill the baby's stomach, reduce appetite at the breast and decrease breastmilk intake – and, consequently, supply. Thus these products are *de facto* breastmilk substitutes. If access to the breast is *un*restricted, babies can stimulate the quantity of breastmilk they need, which can furnish sufficient energy and protein into the second year. The 'nutrient gap' of concern[*] is that of micronutrients[**] iron and zinc. Breastmilk provides a certain amount but total supply depends on the individual baby's birth stores. As these gradually run out, the baby needs to obtain these nutrients from exogenous (ie from outside) sources.

Many foods given to older infants and young children

[*] Vitamin D is also low in breastmilk and is not influenced by the mother's diet during lactation. However a mother's vitamin D intake during pregnancy is vital for her baby's status after birth. Vitamin D is a hormone triggered by sunlight on the skin. This is a geographical and cultural issue.

[**] Micronutrients are the vitamins, minerals and trace elements, as opposed to the macronutrients which are fats, proteins and carbohydrates.

replace a nutritionally superior food, breastmilk, which has disease-protection benefits, with a nutritionally inferior food which may even be a vehicle of infection. A true complementary food would add to the diet nutrients such as iron and zinc, which breastmilk has not evolved to provide in the quantities required by the child who is gradually outgrowing her birth stores. Many so-called complementary foods do not fulfil this function.

There is also the important issue of accustoming* the child to a wide range of foods. Strictly speaking this is not 'complementary' feeding because it does not 'complete' the breastfed child's diet, but is merely the process of learning to eat foods other than milk. But for the purposes of this book the process can be included within our understanding of complementary feeding.

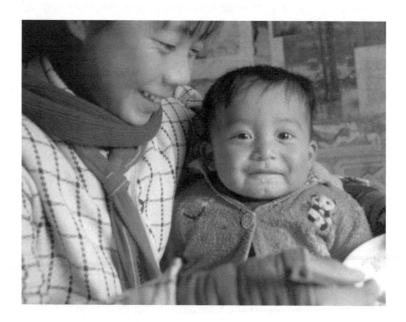

---

* The word 'wean' is derived from an old English word meaning 'to accustom'. The word weaning is not used because inconsistent interpretation causes confusion. The word is used to describe the introduction of solid foods or the cessation of breastfeeding or the transition from breast to artificial feeding. For this reason both WHO and UNICEF avoid this term in their materials to prevent ambiguity.

6

POLITICS

The very concept that one group of human beings should impose their food customs and beliefs on others, or dismiss their child-feeding practices as inadequate, is questionable and can lead to unforeseen consequences. In the early and mid-20th century, before commercial promotion reached its current sophistication, European health professionals in the colonies discouraged women from breastfeeding into the second year and beyond. They thus unwittingly increased malnutrition and death. Health professionals also frowned upon fermented foods, thinking them unhygienic, when in fact the fermentation process suppresses pathogens and enhances nutritional content, including iron bioavailability. These messages undermined beneficial traditional practices.

In recent decades the power and influence of the food industry has increased dramatically.[1] Today, even many privileged human beings seem to believe that they cannot prepare their own children's food, that it must be made in a factory and that they must consult a health professional about how to feed their children. This is astounding if you consider that other higher primates select appropriate foods for their young and teach them how to eat by example.[2] The need for 'scientific' authority to intrude into our personal eating decisions has arisen because food environments have changed rapidly and drastically during the 20th century. This statement is not to glorify the past; bouts of hunger or nutrient deficiency have been part of the human condition for millennia. Famines caused by drought and other natural disasters have always occurred. But hunger and food shortages have often been caused by human intervention, political decisions and economic inequality.[3] Nevertheless, in order to reflect on our topic we must take the long view: the very success of humans as a species shows that we learned how to eat and how to feed our children long before either the formal science of nutrition or modern communications media existed.

Article 24 of The Convention on the Rights of the Child (CRC)[4] refers to the *"provision of adequate nutritious foods and clean drinking water"* but avoids specifying how this is to be achieved. It does not mention that the lack of access to water and nutritious food may be due to processes of 'development'. During the 20th and 21st centuries, thousands of hectares of food-providing land and forest have been appropriated for non-food production (or food for export) and water sources have been contaminated for industrialisation purposes.[*] Research in rural areas of Africa found that sometimes children were better fed during economic downturns.[5] High prices for cash crops often tempt subsistence farmers to divert more land for that crop. This has led to the need for food aid in fertile self-sufficient regions.[6] Wangari Maathai's statement quoted at the beginning of this book describes a process which damages nutrition. Ironically, the cash crop, tea, which has replaced the food crops of her childhood, is an anti-nutrient. Its consumption with food inhibits the absorption of iron in the diet (See Appendix II). Tea drinking with meals contributes to iron-deficiency anaemia (IDA) in women, infants and children and its cultivation takes fertile areas out of food production.[**]

In common with many others, my vision is of a world where there is egalitarian food security for all; where the majority of

---

[*] For example: during the 1990s the Ogoni people of Nigeria protested against the activities of the Shell oil company on their land. The crushing of this protest, with the connivance of the Nigerian government, led to 2,000 deaths and the displacement of 80,000 people. (Kupfer D. Worldwide Shell Boycott. *The Progressive* 1996.)

[**] This does not mean that tea is bad for healthy adults, indeed it has health advantages, but it is ironic that it is cultivated in areas of the world where women and children are undernourished owing to lack of access and entitlement to nutritious food.

humans get their nutrients from their food (and sunshine); where unbiased public education ensures that families have the knowledge and skills to feed their children without the need for different or specially made foods and where government policies protect public health before private profit. Many publications addressing child undernutrition ignore the underlying causes of the injustices that provoke it. They may go into great technical detail about the nutritional content of the diet, but often with the underlying assumption that a mass-produced factory-made food is the way to deal with the problem. Funding may only be available for technical solutions.

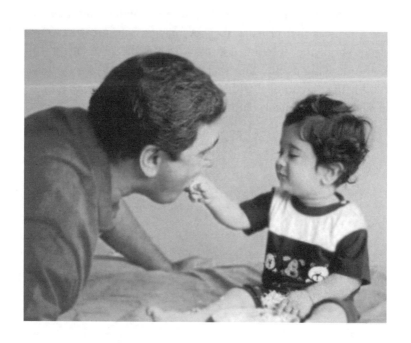

7

NUTRITION

Nutrition is the most inexact of sciences. There are no absolute truths and no perfect diets; the firm convictions of one decade can be superseded in the next. For example, sugar was viewed as a super-food in the 19th century and, when added to the diet of poor families who struggled to meet their energy needs, it saved lives. It also conserved vitamin C-rich fruits for the winter, thus keeping scurvy at bay. It is now a key villain in the obesity pandemic and is implicated in epidemics of dental caries in both poor and rich societies.[1] However, though micronutrient poor (it lacks vitamins and minerals), sugar can still be useful in certain circumstances.

In the 20th century meat was seen as a super-food. Its overconsumption is now implicated in the chronic diseases of affluence, yet if included in complementary feeding it could do much to combat iron-deficiency anaemia. High intakes of red and processed meat are associated with increased deaths from cancer and cardiovascular disease in adults.[2] Most meat is eaten by adult men[3] who, as a group, need fewer of the nutrients in meat than children and women in their reproductive years. In most rich regions meat is eaten almost every day. This is not only unnecessary but disadvantageous to health. Many of these meat consumers would benefit from reduced meat intake.

We must highlight the importance of pleasure in eating. This is not just to do with taste and skilled cooking but the company and affection involved. When humans eat together their oxytocin levels increase and the digestion and metabolism of their food becomes more efficient. A child sitting on the lap of a mother or a relative who loves him may actually utilise his food better because digestive hormones are influenced by oxytocin secretion.[4] The pride and joy that a family takes in food preparation and meal sharing is as important for children as it is for adults. Breastfeeding is a pleasure for a child; eating should be too.

No stance in nutrition is simple. Even popular definitions are unreliable. Foods are classified too roughly and the conventional perceptions of 'protein', 'carbohydrate' or 'fat' foods are misguided. All grains contain protein (sufficient for a balanced diet) yet are classed as carbohydrate foods. Beans, often classed as protein foods, contain carbohydrates; other 'protein foods', such as many meats and cheeses, are predominantly fat foods. During the 1960s a considerable amount of time and money was spent worrying about the supposed global 'protein gap'. Nutritionists stretched their brains to find ways to overcome this. There was even a UN body to deal with the problem.[5] Then someone had the bright idea of redoing the calculations and they found that a 'protein gap' did not exist.[6] Protein is still overemphasised in popular perception. No adult need worry about being protein deficient if she or he eats a diverse diet, even if they never eat any so-called protein food.

We also need to be aware that Recommended Daily Allowances (RDAs) of nutrients, which are set by committees of experts, are not absolute truths. Even the experts themselves admit this.[7]

Some groups of people may be genetically predisposed not to metabolise certain foods,* so a 'healthy' and useful food for one group may harm another. Nevertheless, the extraordinary trait of the human species, shared with pigs, rats and cockroaches, is the ability to survive and thrive on a broad range of diets. We are omnivores. An Inuit (or other indigenous inhabitant of the Arctic regions) living almost exclusively on sea mammals and fish may never eat a vegetable in her life. South Asian or European vegetarians may never eat a scrap of meat or fish. If

---

* For example: favism is a genetic trait common in ethnic groups of the Mediterranean region. People with favism lack the enzyme to digest certain beans (fava beans or *Vicia faba*). Their consumption can lead to acute haemolytic anaemia, which can even affect an exclusively breastfed baby if her mother eats the beans.

they are healthy then they eat a 'healthy' diet. Their group's adaptation to their environmental resources is the reason they have survived, and even flourished, in their particular region. For most diets there is a 'swings and roundabouts' benefit and cost. The traditional Inuit diet, rich in omega-3 fatty acids, is protective against cardiovascular disease so an Inuit is unlikely to suffer a thrombosis due to a blood clot. However, she has a risk of excessive bleeding after an injury because her blood can be slow to clot.[8] The high fibre levels and complex carbohydrates in a traditional South Asian diet protect against cardiovascular disease and bowel cancer but the low quantities of haem iron (ie iron from flesh sources) make women and children more vulnerable to iron-deficiency anaemia. The 'western' diet has become increasingly energy dense, despite fewer people being physically active, to the detriment of health. All these issues are relevant to children's diets, which in essence are very slightly adapted forms of the adult diet. There is no need for 'baby food' for the normal healthy child.

Nutritionists have often got things wrong, even without influence from the food industry. In the 20th century the focus in infant and young child feeding was on increasing the energy density of the diet by adding oil, fat or sugar to the traditional starchy staple because nutritionists had calculated energy and protein 'gaps'.* This was because the traditional starchy staple porridge, made with water, provided a low-energy, high-volume food that filled a child's stomach without providing enough energy and protein to meet her needs. Macronutrient (ie energy and protein) needs had been overestimated because nutritionists had ignored the energy and protein contribution to the diet from breastmilk. If the child was getting enough energy already then adding oil, fat or sugar to increase the energy content diluted the density of micronutrients (ie minerals and vitamins) in the

---

* Cereals provide sufficient protein in relation to energy as a staple diet. In some regions the starchy staple is cassava or manioc (*Manihot utilissima*), a starchy root. This does not contain sufficient protein to meet the needs of a growing child.

food.[9] Nutritionists also urged frequent feeding with the enriched starchy staple porridges. This had the deleterious effect of reducing the frequency of breastfeeds. If you keep urging a young child to eat maize porridge with added oil and sugar, he will not feel hungry enough to ask for the breast or to suckle effectively if offered it. This reduction in stimulus will reduce the quantity of breastmilk – a perfect way to replace the superior food with an inferior one. [I will discuss the focus on cereals later.]

Most inadequate complementary feeding occurs in food-insecure environments. But infants and young children in industrialised societies also suffer inappropriate feeding. They are of course much less likely to die or become stunted in height than children who live in poverty. However, in the late 20th century a new problem of malnutrition emerged, that of overweight and obesity. This problem is now prevalent in poor countries too, creating what has been termed *"the double burden of malnutrition"*.[10]

It may be that inappropriate complementary feeding is more significant in the obesity pandemic than whether a child is breastfed or not. Breastfed infants are rarely obese. If they are, the cause is usually the early addition of solid foods.[11] Infants who stop breastfeeding early (ie before four months) and are given solid foods are more likely to be obese by three years than those who are not, as are children who are formula fed from birth.[12]

This is not only because of the differences between breastmilk and artificial milks. There is evidence that bottle-fed children can lose their ability to self-regulate their appetites, so that infants who are bottle-fed with expressed breastmilk have a disadvantage compared with those who breastfeed. When there is baby-led feeding, the baby's appetite is finely tuned to match his nutritional needs. A breastfed baby who has taken all the milk he requires, both in quantity and content, will spontaneously stop feeding, even if there is still milk in the breast. Bottle-fed babies are far more likely to drain the bottle or cup later on than those who were breastfed.[13]

One of the major, lifelong problems for obese children and

adults is appetite control, something which is established early in life. This raises another risk of RUTFs and RUSFs. They are both energy-dense foods which are appropriate for severely malnourished children. But if they are overprescribed as is already feared, then children with adequate weights may be at risk of obesity. The problem with energy-dense foods has been well explained. The theory is that when there is 'hidden energy', such as happens with high-fat, high-sugar, high-calorie 'fast food', there is passive overconsumption. A typical hamburger meal contains 65% more energy than the average British meal. British nutritionists Prentice and Jebb state that this type of diet *"challenges the human appetite control system"*.[14]

In today's world, two billion people are hungry and one billion people eat too much. How they eat is established when they are babies. It would be disastrous if the attempt to solve the problem of the inadequate feeding of infants and young children resulted in the spread of overweight and obesity. Sadly, there are signs that this is happening.

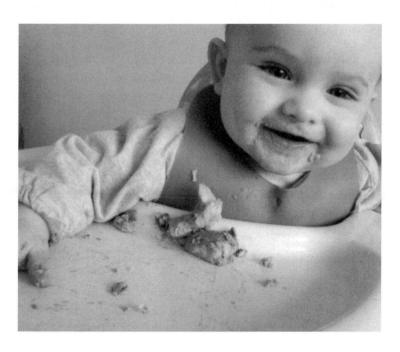

KEY POINTS FROM PART ONE

- This book is not prescriptive but intended to stimulate thought.

- Successful child feeding has been achieved without the intervention of experts.

- Food and water entitlement and availability are crucial.

- The safety of water for drinking is not as important a factor in health as consistent supplies of adequate quantities.

- Complementary feeding is as much about acculturation as physical development.

- Complementary foods often become breastmilk substitutes.

- The promotion of Ready-to-Use Therapeutic Foods (RUTFs), designed to treat severe malnutrition in the context of emergencies, may have negative consequences in non-emergency conditions.

- Nutrition is an inexact science.

- Political decisions affect nutrition.

- Both poor and rich children may be inappropriately fed.

- 'Baby food' is unnecessary.

PART TWO

A CLOSER LOOK

8

FOOD AND NUTRITION:
A HISTORICAL PERSPECTIVE

To reflect on our topic we must ask the following questions:

- What is the 'natural' diet of small children?
- Why do many policy makers and nutritionists endorse the creation of special foods for infants and young children when for the greater part of human existence they ate the same foods as adults?
- Were our ancestors' children at greater risk of malnutrition than our own?

Archaeological scientists have discovered much about early humans' food supplies and eating practices. Humans were living (and using tools) around 100,000 years ago.* Of the 80 billion humans who have walked this earth, 90% have been hunter-gatherers.[1] Relative to human time on earth, farming and agriculture is very new, around 10,000 to 12,000 years old, and dairying a little younger. Industrial society is a mere 200 to 300 years old. In the gradual transition from hunting and gathering to farming there existed what archaeological scientist Martin Jones calls "*multi-track food webs*". These food systems included some cultivation existing alongside hunting, gathering, foraging and fishing, sometimes by different groups, sometimes not.[2] Even after agriculture and pastoralism began to dominate production, these other activities continued and today, practices such as fungi and berry gathering, fishing and collecting molluscs echo our ancestors' survival skills.

---

*   I refer to modern humans (*Homo sapiens*) and not other early hominids such as *Homo erectus*.

9

EVOLUTION AND FOOD SYSTEMS

Humans evolved to eat a diverse diet and multi-track food webs provided these. Diverse diets are associated with reduced disease and mortality.[1] Farming only, or industrialised food only, can cause nutrition problems. We can see examples of multi-track food webs today which include industrialised foods. For example, financially secure, highly educated Europeans may eat a mixture of farmed (grains, meats, vegetables, fruits and fish), foraged (wild fungi, berries, land, river and sea molluscs), hunted (wild mammals, birds and fish) and industrially processed foods (wheat ground into flour and made into bread outside the home).

During the past 100 or so years there has been an accelerating trend towards the use of industrialised food products and food systems. Some have been beneficial. For example iodine deficiency, a 'natural' dietary deficiency, is endemic in certain geographical regions.* This was (and continues to be) overcome through salt iodisation or trade in preserved foods from non-iodine-deficient regions.** Some industrially processed foods play

---

*   Iodine deficiency is exacerbated by environmental degradation, for example when logging leads to erosion and the leaching of soils. Also, ancient beneficial customs may be abandoned. In Papua New Guinea dietary salt used to come from volcanic rock pools. Salt trading with non-iodised salt led to endemic iodine deficiency. This situation was reversed after legislation banning the trading of non–iodised salt. See publications of Peter Pharoah.

** The Himalayas, Alps, US Great Lake Region, Andes and other mountainous regions not covered by sea water during the ice age lack iodine in soils. Populations suffer endemic iodine deficiency (ID) resulting in a high prevalence of goitres, cretinism and lowered intelligence. ID also occurs in riverine areas where seasonal flooding washes away soil. Deficiency can be exacerbated by goitrogens in food plants such as cassava or millet. Logging

a useful role in a 21st-century multi-track food webs.* It is when they are inappropriately promoted and marketed, and suppress other food production and use, that they can have adverse effects on diets.

It is of interest that 'brands' came into being in the 19th century to protect the public from contaminated, adulterated or falsely described food. Cheating our fellow human beings existed long before industrialisation. Watering the milk or making bread with contaminated flour goes back to ancient times.[2] Brands were established to indicate trust in product quality because the buyer could trace the provider. However the current use of brand power by big food corporations is not driven by the quest to improve nutrition but to manipulate the psychological perceptions of the consumer in order to maximise profits. That initial trust of the 'brand' has been exploited to extremes and has become a worshipped marketing tool.

Nevertheless not all industrialised food is bad and not all 'natural' food is good.** Certain foods require highly technical processes to make them edible. For example the burning off of the hard outer casing of the cashew nut (cashew paste is a good food for young children) releases cyanide compounds and is safer and easier to carry out in a factory than in the domestic environment. Cocoa beans (rich in iron, calcium and vitamin A) are difficult to process at household level. Canned fish has a key role to play in combating iodine deficiency and is nutrient-dense.

---

and other soil-eroding activities are also implicated. Salt iodisation has been a successful strategy for addressing this 'natural' problem. For more information see ICCIDD website www.iccidd.org/index.php

*   Eg canned fish can dramatically improve and diversify inland region diets and is especially appropriate for infants and young children.

**   Many plants contain poisons, some edible in certain conditions, eg underripe ackee fruit is poisonous, the ripe fruit is not. Eating the *Lathyrus sativus* pea causes lathyrism, resulting in muscle cramps, weakness or paraplegia. This occurs in Central India and Ethiopia. Also, nutritious animals can become poisonous, eg small birds such as quails can eat the poisonous plant hemlock without harm, but if the quail is eaten it can be fatal. Occasional algae 'blooms' in seawater can make hitherto nutritious shellfish poisonous.

The introduction of non-indigenous foodstuffs has often improved nutrition.* Seasonal scurvy was common in medieval Britain until the introduction of the potato from the Americas because, unlike most grain or root staple foods, it contains vitamin C. Imported sugar enabled the conservation of sour summer fruits as jam,** which helped protect against scurvy. It enabled the inedible to become edible. Few could enjoy bitter oranges, acid gooseberries, rhubarb and other sour wild fruits unless sweetened. Wild honey supplies are haphazard and difficult to gather. Domesticated bees often need to be fed with sugar syrup at the end of winter when their honey stores run low. In the past many domestic bee colonies were killed to remove the honey, or simply died at the end of a long, cold winter.***

Food systems have always been dynamic. Different systems work in different environments. In some regions there may have been a trade-off between food security and good nutrition from food. Farming and food storage protected humans from starvation during adverse climate conditions and seasons but monocultures led to nutrient deficiency disease.**** In the 21st century millions of human beings with no access to land and scant food-survival skills survive on industrially processed foods, even though these

---

* The definition of 'indigenous' can be extrapolated from ecological theories which judge that any plant (or animal) introduced after 1500 CE is 'non-indigenous'. Therefore outside the Americas the potato and the tomato are non-indigenous plants. Theory based on Eser U. Ecological and normative fundamentals of value-judgements in nature conservation: the case of non-indigenous plants. In Freese L, ed. *Advances in Human Ecology, Vol. 7.* JAI Press Inc. 1998, pp293-312.
** Jam and other forms of fruit and vegetable conservation have less vitamin C than fresh products.
*** As well as scurvy, marginal vitamin C deficiency remained a problem in Britain up to the 1940s. Potatoes are one of the best starchy staples because of their broad nutrient content and storage qualities. Sour fruits have other benefits, eg marmalade contains traces of calcium, iron and fibre.
****For example, the vitamin B deficiency diseases pellagra and beri-beri were associated with predominant maize and rice diets respectively.

are associated with obesity and its linked diseases.* Both systems can be associated with a deterioration in the quality of nutrition. Despite the welcome resurgence of knowledge of survival skills,[3] most modern people would starve in a forest rich in foods because they lack the skills to access its resources. Subsistence farming, even with a good climate and fertile soil, requires constant gruelling work, and pests can wipe out a staple crop within days. Seasonal hunger just before the harvest is commonplace. In many societies women were (and are) the main food producers and their work burdens are often overwhelming. The departure of men for labour or military service makes a difference to family food production.

Context is everything. An African subsistence farmer may be unable to nourish her children adequately because she lives in an iodine-deficient region and has no cash to buy foodstuffs (eg canned fish) containing iodine. If her staple food is cassava, this exacerbates the risk of iodine deficiency because it contains substances which impede the take-up of iodine in the diet.** Cassava is a poor crop, nutritionally low in protein and energy, but it is drought resistant and easy to grow. Ideally it is a famine food, an insurance against other crop failure, and it is a useful addition to a varied, mixed diet.

A US woman, especially a poor one, may be unable to establish healthy eating habits in her children because she has scant access to diverse fresh foods, lacks the knowledge, skill and time to prepare them, and is exposed to aggressive marketing of industrially produced foods that are high in sugar, salt and/or fat.*** Her child may receive plenty of nutrients to grow rapidly but may develop tastes which predispose him to a lifetime of overweight or obesity. It may be cheaper in terms of access and cost for a poor US woman to buy ready-made packaged or takeaway food than to prepare her own.

---

*   About half the world's population now lives in urban environments.

**   Cassava contains goitrogens, substances which inhibit iodine absorption.

*** Both in the USA and the UK it is often hard to find sources of high-quality fresh foods, especially in poor residential areas.

Better educated and richer Europeans and North Americans have more diverse diets and better health than less-educated and poorer citizens who have a narrower diet. In industrialised countries the greater the inequality the greater the prevalence of overweight and obese children (and adults).[4] US 'fast food' style eating has spread across the world, damaging nutrition and health and the multi-track food webs which have underpinned some of the most balanced diets which are ideal for infants and young children. The cycle of de-skilling and dependency on industrialised products is bad for infants and young children.[5]

10

SALTY, SWEET AND FAT:
THE HUMAN DRIVES FOR TASTE

The innate human drive for nutrient density is ruthlessly exploited by the marketing of industrially processed foods. Most humans seek out salt, sweetness and fat in foods: a desire for saltiness led us to the high mineral content of flesh foods, for sweetness to riper, and therefore more digestible, fruits and for satiation to the energy and nutrient-dense foods such as nuts, seeds and certain parts of animals such as bone marrow. The delight in finding the sweetest honey ant (see Appendix I), the fattiest fish or the 'strongest' tasting morsel was a nutritional advantage for adults and children living in an environment where humans, including young children, had to be active and ingenious in order to gather, forage or hunt their food.[1] In the past toddlers always stayed with the family group and they would have learned their skills early.

II

HUMAN PLUMPNESS

Another innate human survival trait is the laying down of body fat. Only sea mammals equal or exceed the human capacity for fat storage, which provides an energy reserve to survive periods of scarcity. This is one reason why humans are more successful in reproductive terms than other primates. Female humans store more fat than males.* This is why humans (unlike most other land mammals) can maintain a pregnancy and lactate even during times of food shortage.** Plumpness enables children to get through periods of illness. I am not aware of research in this area (and it would be unethical to do) but it may be that the welcome decline in common childhood infections has exacerbated problems of overweight and obesity. Until the latter half of the 20th century, the majority of children suffered inevitable periods of poor appetite (anorexia) and weight loss during bouts of measles, mumps and other infections. We can only rejoice in the life-saving benefits of mass immunisation but may consider that, like TV and motor transport, this may be another factor in the 'obesogenic' environment.[1]

The favouring of plumpness in children and cultural practices to urge them to eat energy-dense foods probably arose because plump children survived infections better than thin children.

---

* Fat is not always visible: a slim woman will still carry more body fat than a man of roughly the same size.

** Many other mammals (eg badgers) will reabsorb the fetus during times of food scarcity. Women have borne infants and lactated successfully in concentration camps, during famines and in other adverse conditions. This does not mean that food deprivation is good for the mother or child but the robustness of human reproduction is amazing. See Prentice AM & Prentice A. Reproduction against the odds. *New Scientist* 1988; 118:42-46.

This custom actually contaminated scientific understanding during the 20th century. The 40-year belief that the greater weights of US children, who were artificially fed and given early complementary foods, were the ideal, has contributed to current childhood nutrition problems.[2]

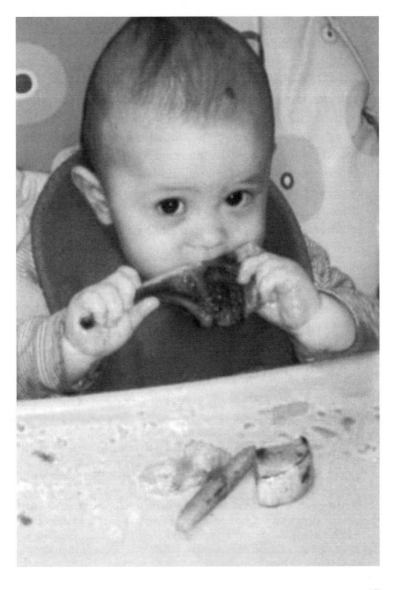

12

THE TIMING OF COMPLEMENTARY FEEDING

It has been deduced from a range of evidence sources that for the greater part of human existence, children breastfed for between four and seven years.[1] The resulting pause in menstruation and ovulation (lactational amenorrhoea)* protected women from the adverse effects of closely spaced pregnancies and, together with a mineral-rich diet, from iron-deficiency anaemia. Good maternal iron status and delayed umbilical cord-cutting would have facilitated good iron stores in infants at birth.[2] Iron and zinc are the crucial nutrients that breastmilk does not provide in adequate amounts in the second year of life (see Appendix II).

Breastfeeding provided food security during drought or other adverse conditions. A child might have alternated between periods of exclusive and non-exclusive breastfeeding during toddlerhood depending on environmental food abundance. It is often still assumed that the main reason for complementary feeding is an insufficient quantity of breastmilk to exclusively feed in the second year but, as has been demonstrated by lifelong wet nurses,** breastmilk quantity waxes and wanes according to the amount of suckling. Complementary food is necessary to fill a (variable) micronutrient 'gap' not (in most cases) an energy and protein gap. Modern social and economic customs and marketing

---

*   Lactational amenorrhoea is the term used to describe the normal physiological state whereby a woman who is lactating does not menstruate or ovulate. It is maintained by frequent, baby-led breastfeeding, including night feeding. See Palmer G. *The Politics of Breastfeeding*. Pinter & Martin 2009, pp136-140.

**   Wet nurses sometimes suckled two or more infants simultaneously and continued professionally to suckle series of infants for several years without adverse effects on the wet nurses' health. See: Palmer G. *The Politics of Breastfeeding*. Pinter & Martin 2009, p186. Also: Fildes V. *Wet-Nursing*. Basil Blackwell 1988.

messages impede women from the frequent and continued breastfeeding long after infancy that would have been the norm for our ancestors.

The use of an age-based cut-off for the introduction of complementary foods is unphysiological and is a clumsy (though perhaps necessary) public health tool. As Gill Rapley has pointed out so cogently, children do not crawl, walk, cut their teeth or talk at an exact age, so why are they all expected to need complementary feeding at the same age? It is only recently in human existence that people have taken age so seriously. In prehistoric times mothers would have responded to infant behaviour. Eating utensils were not used for thousands of years. Why would a breastfeeding mother bother to coax her child to eat something when the breast was always there? [I ask the same question today: why bother?] When a child can sit up, fix his gaze on an object, reach out and grasp it, he will put something edible in his mouth, if food is available. As he gets older, improving dexterity and visual acuity enable him to pick up smaller objects. At the same time his natural maturation of oral development enables him to chew.[3]

Children do not have to be taught to eat; these developmental reflexes are innate. Pureed, semi-liquid and diluted foods are unnecessary, because if a child cannot chew, he is not ready to have anything other than breastmilk (or the best possible breastmilk substitute). These foods (either industrially or home produced), which are customarily given to infants, are *de facto* inferior breastmilk substitutes. Just as some children start to walk at nine and others at eighteen months, so some children might eat earlier or later than others. Some breastfeeding infants are uninterested in foods until the end of the first year or later, while others are already reaching out and grasping food at five months. When investigators followed a group of British babies to see when they reached out to pick up 'finger foods', they found that just over half had reached for food before six months while some were still not reaching out at eight months.[4] All children are different. The six-month edict is a public health guideline, not a description of infant behaviour or normality. The risk is that children with early iron-deficiency anaemia may lack appetite and the energy to reach out and grasp their foods, but this is an issue of cord-cutting protocols, food availability and ignorance (see Appendix II). It is not an innate problem of children but the result of their environment.

There is some evidence that children exposed to a range of 'wholesome and natural' foods will select a healthy balance that meets their nutritional needs.[5] The issue is access to diverse and nutritious foods. Amidst the multi-track food webs, our ancestors' babies and toddlers ate the same food as older children and adults, learning through imitation. Mothers and other family members probably assisted the child at first. Many modern children are provided with 'activity learning' toys to stimulate their cognitive skills. These replace the fascinating lessons of learning how to prize open a mollusc shell or split the hard casing of some fruits. For older infants, mothers and other carers would have selected softer parts of animals, such as marrowbone and brain tissue, and also pre-chewed some harder foods. Passing food directly to the baby from a mother's mouth, known as 'kiss feeding' is still practised by some groups today and may be the origin of romantic/sexual kissing.[6] Most children would have fended for themselves quite quickly. In a food-rich environment many children can do well without being actively fed, though children benefit from a mother or other loving carer who notes whether they are eating or not and shares their own food. However, it may be that the child who did not actively seek out food might have been allowed to die because autonomy and self-sufficiency were important for a group's survival.[7]

13

WHAT DID YOUNG CHILDREN EAT DURING PREHISTORIC TIMES?

Evidence indicates that prehistoric diets were more micronutritient dense than modern diets.* Archaeologist Francis Pryor is confident that the inhabitants of Bronze Age Britain were extremely well nourished. Bone analysis shows uninterrupted growth and no nutrient deficiencies. This indicates that there were no problems with the transition from breastfeeding to an adult diet.[1]

Existing hunter-gatherers whose diets echo those of prehistory do not have modern health problems (eg hypertension, obesity, cardiovascular disease, diabetes), nor their children the usual high rates of gastrointestinal and respiratory infections found in poor regions. Derrick Jelliffe reported that children of the nomadic hunter-gatherer Hadza of Tanzania did not develop the malnutrition or deficiency diseases of the surrounding farmers' children.[2] Most hunter-gatherers were nomadic or semi-nomadic and therefore did not create the reservoirs of disease that settlement induces. Poor environmental hygiene (contaminated water and inadequate faecal disposal systems) and resulting infections contribute to the cycle of child malnutrition. Sick children do not feed well and poorly fed children are more vulnerable to infection. Some specific nutrient deficiencies are linked to the environment as much as to diet. For example, vitamin A deficiency has been directly linked to the absence of sewage disposal systems.[3] This is because frequent diarrhoeal disease damages the intestine, causing nutrient malabsorption.**

---

*   Among many techniques, scientists can discern from bone analysis how long a child was breastfed.

**   Despite the health advantages of the hunter-gatherer lifestyle, throughout

Some nutritional theorists argue that our bodies evolved over thousands of years to cope with entirely different dietary patterns from those of the contemporary industrialised world. The adaptability of humans is one reason why diets vary throughout the world. However, during recent centuries changes in diet and behaviour have happened extremely rapidly. Our bodies are probably still adapted to a time when humans were physically active and ate a spare and varied diet of foods rich in micronutrients.

Older babies and young children would have eaten or been fed parts of small mammals, molluscs, insects and other invertebrates, shellfish and other coastal sea creatures. Nuts, fruits, leaves, shoots, tubers, wild grass seeds and fungi may also have been eaten but the texture and nutrient density of small animals were ideal to fulfil small children's nutritional needs. Breastmilk did not evolve to provide much iron and zinc after the first year or so because it was not necessary.* Just as humans evolved to get their vitamin D from sunshine and not from breastmilk, so they met their early iron and zinc needs from birth stores and then later from sources in their environment (see Appendix II).

the 20th and 21st centuries all governments have at best failed to protect – and at worst persecuted – nomadic and hunter-gatherer modes of living. Most settled peoples patronise or despise the nomadic groups who live in their countries. We have much to learn from them.

*   Breastmilk also does not provide sufficient vitamin D. The term vitamin is a misnomer as vitamin D is a hormone triggered by sunlight. Humans evolved to live out of doors and vitamin D deficiency is more a problem of lifestyle and where you live rather than diet. I do not address this issue in detail in this book.

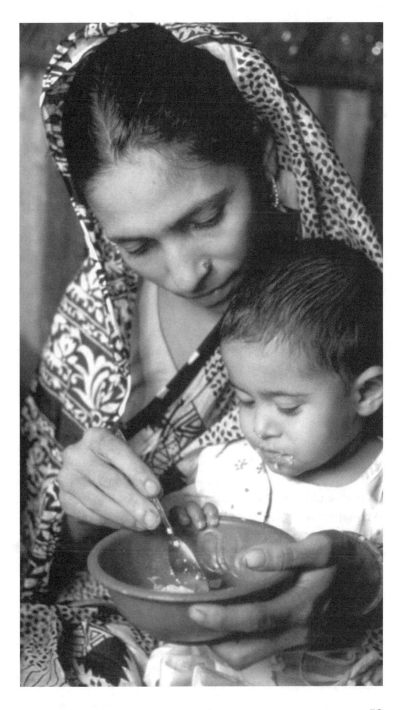

14

ARE CEREALS APPROPRIATE
FOOD FOR BABIES?

Vegetable and fruit purees and cereal porridges were not part of the human diet until relatively recently, that is until around 10,000 years ago.* The very word 'baby food' means a soft, semi-liquid adaptation of an adult food, often cereal based. Infants and young children did not evolve to consume these products as their first foods and there is scientific theory to demonstrate this.[1]

Our ancestors' children were getting iron by scrabbling in the earth (a rich source) and snacking on little creatures (see Appendix II). As described above, infants go through a phase when they instinctively put everything they find on the ground in their mouths. Today's adults are usually horrified, remove the object, replace it with a plastic toy or dummy (pacifier) and try to place the child in a 'safe' environment. However, if you allowed your one-year old to crawl in a garden she might pick up an insect, worm or snail and eat it, together with some soil, without your knowledge.** With some justification, we fear parasites, poisonous insects and plants harming our children. However, humans are social animals and the accumulated knowledge of what was safe or not would have been held and passed on orally by a group familiar with their natural environment. Though parasites (such as hookworm or roundworm) can exacerbate nutrient

---

*   Stone querns for grinding grain have been found and dated to have been made just around the time farming was becoming established 10,000 years ago.

** During the time I wrote this document, my nine-month-old grandson picked up a large garden snail and popped it into his mouth with relish. I removed it for two reasons: one because I was *in loco parentis* and I knew his parents would be upset if I let him eat it; two because I was aware that a London snail might carry pathogens and industrial pollutants.

deficiencies, we have to be aware that being entirely parasite-free may be a trigger of allergy.[2]

The great majority of children living in poverty who do not get enough good food suffer from a lack of many key nutrients. However, in this book I have decided to focus on just one nutrient and use it as an example. I have chosen iron because iron deficiency is a major and unresolved nutrient deficiency of young children.

Iron is best provided by foods of animal origin (flesh foods), and particularly meat and seafood. These foods are rich in the well-absorbed form of iron (haem iron) and enhance the absorption of the less bioavailable form of iron (non-haem) in plant foods, if eaten together. For example, small molluscs are good sources of bioavailable iron. They are also soft (or easily softened) and digestible.

Public health authorities give out ambiguous messages. For example, FAO/WHO states: "*It is possible to meet these high requirements (ie for iron) if the diet has a consistently high content of meat and foods rich in ascorbic acid (vitamin C). In the most developed countries today, infant cereal products are the staple foods for that period of life. Commercial products are regularly fortified with iron and ascorbic acid and they are usually given together with fruit juices and solid foods containing meat, fish and vegetables. The fortification of cereal products with iron and ascorbic acid is important in meeting the high dietary needs, especially considering the importance of optimal iron nutrition during this phase of brain development.*"[3] We have to question why cereals are promoted as the principal food of infants and young children in rich countries when they are naturally low in key nutrients. It may be because of extreme caution or even fear of giving meat and seafood to infants and young children. Popular information promotes fruits and vegetable purees and cereals as the first foods.[4] It is not a question of poverty, because in many industrialised countries even the diets of disadvantaged adults may contain excessive amounts of meat.[*]

I have seen a toddler in Taiwan eating cooked oysters and my Spanish daughter-in-law assumes she ate all these seafoods before she could walk. However, in many regions flesh foods are reserved for older children and adults or only introduced to young children with great caution. In areas where their value for small children is traditionally recognised (such as parts of China), poor people cannot afford them, while the wealthy are increasingly ensnared by marketing to give commercial baby foods based on cereals, overpriced purees of locally available fruits and vegetables or spurious versions of popular dishes 'filled' with starches and thickeners. For example, a complementary food on the UK market contains 'organic sweetcorn and potato'.[5] These vegetables are naturally low in iron and the nutrient is not even mentioned on the label's nutrition information. This product replaces breastmilk or a more nutritious solid food with micronutrient-poor starch.

Most modern babies' and toddlers' first non-milk foods are starchy staples such as rice or other cereal-based porridges, either home-prepared or industrially produced. Some parents give mashed fruits or 'soups'. Despite the progress towards evidence-based public health edicts, I have not come across any challenge to these customs. Official public health messages, commercial advertising and popular perception see rice as a 'gentle' first food, benign and beneficial. In fact, though an excellent basis for the adult diet, for infants and children under two years it is at best a low-nutrient food that accustoms the child to a texture and taste; at worst it replaces breastmilk. It is a breastmilk substitute rather than a complementary food.

The solution to cereal's lack of key nutrients for babies has been to compensate with industrialised fortification of commercially

---

[*] No adult need eat meat more than once a week and reduction of consumption can benefit health. Studies of vegetarians in industrialised countries show certain health advantages. For an overview of the pros and cons of vegetarian diets see: Sanders TAB. Vegetarian Diets. (In: Geissler C & Powers H, eds. *Human Nutrition 11th edition*. Elsevier 2007, pp335-343.)

produced cereal products and to urge their use. Health and nutrition agencies do this through their public health messages as much as the companies do through marketing. Cereal as a staple food is fine for older children and adults but it is inadequate for infants and young children under two.

The key fact to be aware of in this discussion is that starch is the major component of cereals and the enzyme amylase is needed to digest this. Babies do not develop the enzyme amylase in adequate quantities for the digestion of starch until they are two years old and over.

What can be said about this situation? Many people, and not just vegetarians, are worried at the idea of giving a six-month old a flesh product. Yet biologically it is more appropriate for meeting a baby's nutritional needs beyond breastmilk. Breastmilk actually contains some amylase but cows' milk and infant formulas do not. Its purpose in breastmilk is unclear but it may act as an antibacterial factor degrading bacterial cell walls.[6] Alert readers may consider that this amylase is an evolutionary adaptation to the practice of feeding babies with cereals and that breastfeeding might aid their digestion. However, there is insufficient amylase in breastmilk to break down the starch in a cereal meal.

Cereals can have other adverse effects. The Ethiopian grain, teff, is exceptionally high in iron but most cereals, particularly rice, wheat and maize, are low in this key nutrient. The minerals and vitamins predominate in the outer part of the cereal grain (the husk), which babies cannot digest. This husk also contains phytates which prevent the absorption of important minerals such as iron, zinc and calcium. Phytates strongly inhibit iron absorption.[*] The husk provides fibre, which is protective against bowel cancer and other adult diseases, but babies and toddlers do not need this fibre and cannot digest it. To combat this

---

[*]   Excess iron in the diet can be dangerous so there is a useful role for phytates. Iron overload is a serious medical condition and is more common in men. Wholegrain diets are beneficial for most older children and adults and are protective against some chronic diseases such as cardiovascular disease and bowel cancer.

indigestibility the husk is removed. This age-old practice was not due to awareness of the effects of phytates but because human societies favoured the 'whiteness' of refined cereals for cultural reasons. The word 'wheat' is related to 'white' and many societies associate whiteness with 'purity' and quality.*

Modern industrialised society has addressed the problem of the widespread practice of feeding babies the 'wrong food' by fortifying dehusked cereals with the minerals and vitamins removed in the refining process. Whatever our feelings about the food industry, this compromise of refinement, followed by enrichment, has provided children with a more nutritious foodstuff than the polished, dehusked cereal that many adults favour. Parboiling of rice before dehusking makes some B vitamins 'stick' to the inner part of the grain although minerals in the husk are lost.**

Certain cereals contain the 'toxic protein' gluten. It is present in wheat, barley, rye and oats but not in maize, millet or rice.*** Gluten intolerance (coeliac disease) is a common genetic disease in the western world, affecting between one in 130 to one in 500 of the population in Europe and one in 133 in the USA. The gluten damages the mucosa of the small intestine and affects nutrient absorption.[7] Early introduction of gluten-containing cereals to infants may also be a factor in type 1 diabetes.[8]

Long before industrialisation, societies devised processing methods which by chance (or natural selection) enhanced the nutritional value of cereals. The ancient peoples of Central America made tortillas with maize processed with lime (the mineral not the fruit). This made the amino acid tryptophan**** and

---

*   Martin Jones in *Feast* states that barley is hardier, more adaptable to difficult climates and contains higher levels of nutrients than wheat. *Feast: Why humans share food.* Oxford University Press, 2007.

**   Parboiling is both ancient and modern. It probably originated in India 2,000 to 4,000 years ago. It is now a common method of factory processing. (See: Owen S. *The Rice Book.* Frances Lincoln, 1988.)

*** Millet does not contain gluten and has higher levels of iron and calcium than wheat or rice, but it contains goitrogens which can exacerbate iodine deficiency.

**** An amino acid is an organic compound. Tryptophan is an essential amino

the B vitamin niacin bioavailable. Maize was taken to Europe, Africa and North America without learning these techniques and pellagra (niacin deficiency) became widespread in regions where maize became the staple food.

Fermentation is another ancient process which enhances vitamin content, destroys phytates, makes iron more bioavailable and improves digestibility.[9] The microorganisms or enzymes that cause the biological changes overwhelm pathogens and render foods safe for storage without refrigeration. The leavening process of yeasted breads (as opposed to unleavened flat breads) destroys or reduces the intrinsic phytates which inhibit iron absorption. Yoghurt and other fermented milk products are safer than fresh milk, and fermented vegetables such as German sauerkraut and Korean kimchee are micronutrient rich and anti-pathogenic.[*]

Our current knowledge of cereals indicates that it is scientifically illogical to endorse the convention that a child's first food in addition to breastfeeding must be a cereal-based soft food. It is merely culturally and commercially expedient.

---

acid meaning that it cannot be synthesised in the body and therefore must be available in the diet. Proteins are made up of chains of amino acids.

[*] During the 20th century droves of well-intentioned health professionals told traditional societies to stop giving fermented foods to children, claiming that they were unhygienic. The contrary is true. In the absence of refrigeration (which applies to the majority of human beings in poverty) fermented foods are safer and more nutritious than foods processed in other ways.

15

A WORD ABOUT ANIMAL MILK

Though low in iron, animal milk can be a useful food and provide a range of nutrients. Until around 10,000 years ago, animal milk was not used as a food so it is a relatively new food product for human society. After early childhood, most humans do not produce the stomach enzyme lactase to digest milk sugar (lactose). However, this does not mean that animal milk and its processed products (fermented milks, yoghurts, cheeses, butter etc) are bad for everyone. Northern Europeans and other pastoralist groups developed the mutation of producing lactase after early childhood and so could digest animal milk into adulthood. Probably because of European cultural dominance, the normal human trait (of not producing lactase) is now described as 'alactasia', as though it is abnormal. People with 'alactasia' get pain, wind and flatulence if they drink fresh milk. The 20th-century worship of milk has been so great that products have been developed to add to milk so that adults can digest the lactose in cows' milk. This is unnecessary for health because all the nutrients in milk can be found in other foods. The African-Americans, Asians and other groups who are genetically predisposed not to drink milk are the 'normal' human beings. Northern Europeans have a mutation in that their infant digestive process persists into adulthood. Fresh milk drinking has not been wholly beneficial.[1*] The fact is that the mutant Europeans have been such colonisers and busybodies that they have spread their habits to the whole world: good for some but not for all.

In the modern world cows' milk is perceived not just as a useful

---

*   Before the advent of pasteurisation and refrigeration milk drinking was a risky practice. In the UK, bovine TB from drinking infected milk caused over 800,000 deaths between 1850 and 1950. Brucellosis can also be transmitted from animals to humans through milk consumption.

food for infants and young children but absolutely essential for almost everyone. Governments and international agencies have invested millions in supporting the powerful dairy industries, sometimes crushing small local producers. In common with a wide range of foods, milk can play a useful role in a mixed diet, but possible negative effects are not always considered.[*] Epidemiological studies have shown an association between milk intake and prevalence of iron deficiency.[2] Uniquely among animal protein sources it appears to stimulate insulin-like growth factor (IGF-1) secretion and promote growth in the child.[3] Whether this has adverse side effects is not known. One hypothesis suggests that early contact with cows' milk may be implicated in breast cancer in later life.[4] Some studies have linked early contact with cows' milk-based products to the incidence of type 1 diabetes.[5] Many commercial complementary foods contain powdered cows' milk, which may contain intrinsic pathogens.[6]

We also know that modern dairy industries use methods whose safety is unproven. Synthetic bovine somatotrophin hormone (used to increase milk yield) is banned in Europe yet routinely used in US milk production. The use of antibiotics and other veterinary products may be unsafe. The serious and accelerating problem of antibiotic resistance in pathogens which affect humans may be connected with antibiotic use in animal husbandry, including the dairy industry.[7] There are also sporadic or systemised contamination cases such as the 2008 Sanlu scandal in China, where cows' milk used for infant formula manufacture was contaminated at source.[8] The focus of concern was, quite properly, on damaged artificially fed infants but it is likely that the same milk was used for other products for young children and that adverse effects were not sought or recognised. Monitoring of these products and their effects is inadequate. Most research on complementary feeding takes place in developing countries; in

---

[*]   I leave aside the major issue of the effects on breastfeeding of cows' milk product promotion and breastmilk substitute marketing in this book. I have covered this issue in *The Politics of Breastfeeding* (Palmer G. Pinter & Martin 2009.)

industrialised countries there is an assumption that products are benign but there is little official scrutiny of foods for infants and young children unless an adverse event occurs and is documented.

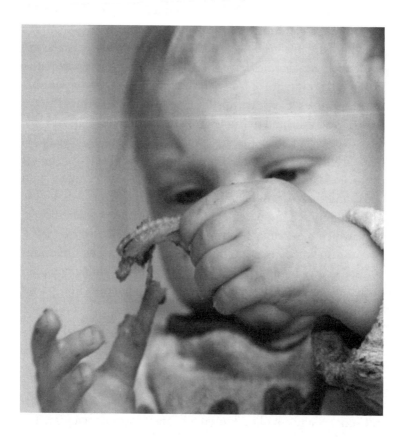

16

WHY DON'T WE GIVE OUR BABIES MOLLUSCS AND INSECTS?

If they are so rich in the key nutrients for babies why do we commonly avoid oysters, other molluscs and seafoods as complementary foods? They are nutrient-dense and easy to swallow and digest. Little ones come in baby bite-sized portions, exactly like the small toys that infants love putting in their mouths. There are some valid reasons. As human populations became more settled and more densely populated, seashores became polluted with human faeces, and consequently oral-faecal pathogens transmitted infections (and killed) through seafood. Such pathogens thrive in hotter climates. This may be why certain religious and cultural groups forbade the consumption of such foods. In the 20th century, the same seafoods have been vulnerable to the health hazard of industrial contamination. Nevertheless, where vigilant health and safety supervision is practised, these products provide safe, nutrient-dense and popular foods for the rich. They may be a hard currency earner in a developing country. For example, in parts of Asia, the lucrative prawn industry exports to rich countries from regions where many young children have inadequate diets and where both companies and health authorities may promote commercial cereals and milks for infants and young children.[1]

Many early humans lived in settlements by the sea and left vast heaps of shells. Nutrition scientist Michael Crawford postulates that humans evolved in coastal areas because a diet based on sea products contains the ideal fatty acids (and iodine) for optimum brain development. Some lake dwellers have similar nutritional advantage because some of the large lakes are actually landlocked ancient seas.[2]

Whether they have access to the sea or not, most hunter-gatherers eat diets of great diversity, and diverse diets are associated with better nutrition.[3] The customary diet of the !Kung of the Kalahari Desert in Southern Africa consisted of eighty-five species of food plant, including thirty roots and bulbs. They consumed fifty-four species of animals.[4] The full-term baby of such a nomadic mother would be born with good iron stores. His mother would have sufficient iron because of her diet, well-spaced births (three or four years) due to continued frequent breastfeeding, and minimal episodes of menstruation. She would have had her first period (menarche) much later than is normal in industrialised societies, probably because she would never have been overweight.* It is unlikely that the umbilical cord would be cut too soon, as is the norm in most modern healthcare settings, so the baby would get his rightful amount of iron via blood transferred from the placenta.[5]

Insects (and insect products) provide a significant source of nutrient-dense foods. They have always been part of the human diet (see Appendix I). Currently 1,509 species of insects are eaten by 3,000 ethnic groups across 120 countries.[6] Many would be (and may be) ideal additions to the diet of the infant and young child. Various species are favoured as seasonal treats and may be traded. Many people deny that they eat insects because they do not perceive particular food products as insects. For example, in China, silk worm pupae are a delicacy but consumers do not think of themselves as insect eaters. In the same way, most consumers of dairy products would deny drinking animal body fluids or eating mould, yet they drink milk and eat cheese. It is cultural bias not lack of nutritional value that deters endorsement and promotion of insect use. The next section addresses this issue.

---

* The age of menarche is strongly related to body size and body fat.

17

CULTURAL AND RELIGIOUS BELIEFS

I am aware that already some readers must be recoiling in horror at the idea of giving anyone, let alone a baby, a shellfish or an insect, because in their religion or culture these are proscribed foods and such is the success of cultural communication that members of that group feel disgust at the thought of eating them. Every single human group, whether ethnic, religious, philosophical, cultural, class or caste, has food taboos, and the rationales for maintaining them overlap. For example, many vegetarians' and vegans' eating practices are based on moral principles (ie it is wrong to kill),* but most also believe that their health is better for such practices. And this may be true, because what we believe about something may influence our bodies. The placebo effect of pills which contain no drug, surgery where nothing is done or a benign medical ritual is known to have measurable effects on many individuals.[1] There may be a similar effect with food. Certainly we know that if someone eats and enjoys a food and is then told that it contains something that is taboo, he may feel disgusted or even vomit. Parents influence their children's disgust or pleasure over individual foods by expressing their own reactions.

During the 20th century, simultaneously in the USA and the USSR, propaganda overvalued the health-giving properties of meat and cows' milk, as much because of political and economic interests and ideologies, as contemporary nutritionists' miscalculations about protein requirements.[2] There is not space here to discuss all the nutritional effects of food taboos but it is relevant to be aware that, even in prehistoric times, groups would

---

*   For a scholarly account of the influence of Indian vegetarianism during the European age of enlightenment see: Stuart T. *The Bloodless Revolution: radical vegetarians and the discovery of India*. Harper Press, 2006.

refrain from eating certain locally available foods for reasons of cultural beliefs and identity.[3]

Humans have a strong drive to belong to a group, and identification with that group is linked to shared eating practices. Food taboos help people to feel they are different from, or even superior to, the next group. Even the omnivorous Shanghainese will say, *"We are not like the Hong Kong people, we would never eat a cat"*. I think of myself as infinitely omnivorous but I have taboos against eating a hamburger or a product produced by Nestlé. My feelings about these products may echo those of a Muslim who will avoid non-halal meat. We both believe the products have been prepared in an unclean way. For me the uncleanliness is moral and concerns production methods and marketing behaviours. Both of us feel upset if our children eat these products.

Whether people do or do not eat cats in Hong Kong (after all, meat is meat whichever animal it comes from), or I eat a Nestlé chocolate product (chocolate is chocolate), is irrelevant. How people feel about a food affects human society profoundly. In India, poor people eat more millet than rice. Millet contains more useful nutrients than rice* and grows better in drought-ridden areas. The first change that a poor family makes after a small rise in income is to abandon millet as their staple food and change to rice. This move to a less nutritionally advantageous staple occurs in many societies. Richer consumers of rice can compensate by eating nutritious accompanying foods and hence contrive a good balanced diet. Poor people often cannot afford this. 'Whiteness' may still be a key factor. In Europe and the USA poor people favour white over brown bread and in Africa white maize meal is favoured over yellow.

It seems that human groups have for thousands of years identified themselves and each other by what they do and do not eat. This affects how children are fed. Marketing hooks into our sense of identity. Millions of Chinese who know how

---

*   Millet has higher levels of calcium and iron than wheat or rice and is gluten free.

to prepare nutritious and delicious meals, ideal for infants and young children, are seduced by the marketing of industrialised foods for their offspring because as aspirational parents they believe that feeding their children the food of rich westerners will give advantages. Noticing so many overweight boys, I said to a Chinese friend: *"They'll have heart disease by 40"*, she replied, *"My mother-in-law criticises me because my sons don't look like that."*

Food is not just a way of keeping our bodies going, it has great significance for our identities. Many believe that their souls will be damaged if they eat a proscribed food or if they do not eat a food of great symbolic importance. Theories of hot and cold, clean and unclean, correct and incorrect foods go back to ancient times and have great significance within cultures. When health workers tell vegan parents that they must give their children animal foods, they are insulting their beliefs and trampling on their identities. It can be the same when they urge families not to give rice or honey to a newborn.

Conservatism and fear of the unknown also plays a part. In the 17th century, English Pilgrim Fathers arrived at Cape Cod in North America not knowing how to fish, hunt or farm. Although extremely hungry they would not eat the abundant lobsters or molluscs on the beach.[4] Folk memories create taboos. The Irish long despised seafood because its consumption was associated with the 19th-century famines. Ireland's surrounding seas are rich in these products but the bulk are exported to Spain and France, whose citizens pay high prices for products they consider to be healthy, delicious and luxurious.

Some theorists call the early historical change of diet from diverse wild products to planted crops 'cerealisation', and see it as a cause of the deterioration in human health and stature.[5] The opposite argument is that without cereals as staple foods, human populations could not have expanded so much. Currently, the rich industrialised populations are using up more than their fair share of nutrient-dense foods while the poor have insufficient. The broad consensus among nutritionists is that for the majority of adults, a diverse plant-based diet is desirable, that vegetarianism is a healthy option, and that non-vegetarians should eat animal foods sparingly. In the modern diet, the customary proportions of allocation of food types for adults and children seem to be the wrong way round. Adults need a lower and children a higher proportion of animal foods. Modern irrational taboos and cultural beliefs about complementary feeding impede good child nutrition.

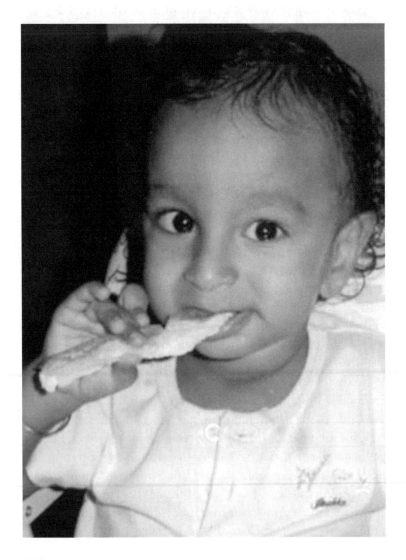

KEY POINTS FROM PART TWO

- For most of human existence, everyone, including older infants and young children, ate diverse, nutrient-dense foods. These were available through systems which archaeological scientists call 'multi-track food webs'.

- For most of human existence, a child would have breastfed for four to seven years. This would have ensured nutrient security during scarcity.

- Food systems are dynamic and women are usually the main producers and processors.

- Humans have innate drives to favour certain food tastes and a capacity for body fat storage that exceeds any other land mammal. These traits favoured survival of the human species.

- A diverse diet is best.

- Some industrially processed foods are useful and some 'natural' foods harmful; the introduction of non-indigenous foods can be an advantage.

- Iron deficiency is a major global health problem of older infants and young children that is associated with predominantly cereal diets.

- Clamping the umbilical cord too soon after birth is a cause of iron deficiency in infants and young children.

- Children may not be physiologically ready to digest cereals until around two years of age. Gluten, found in some cereals, is harmful in certain populations.

- Older infants and young children can digest flesh foods.

- Small animals, including seafood, molluscs and insect foods, could add nutrient density to the diets of young children.

- Dependency on industrially processed foods and the destruction of food production and preparation skills create nutrition problems.

PART THREE
PROCESSES FOR CHANGE

18

THE LANGUAGE OF FOOD

This book is based on a paper written for the International Baby Food Action Network (IBFAN), whose main concern is to halt the abuse and exploitation of parents and carers by companies who manufacture and promote industrially produced breastmilk substitutes and other foods for babies and young children. These foods in themselves may or may not be appropriate. They may reduce women's domestic work burdens but may also create dependency and long-term food insecurity. Part of the strategy of protest is to promote the use of foods from non-industrialised sources. Common words and phrases used in these statements include: *fresh, home-prepared, indigenous, local, locally produced, natural, wholesome, traditional* and *unprocessed*. Many are blithely used in the literature without definition. This is a pity. Decades of research comparing breastfeeding with artificial feeding were wasted because researchers neglected to define their terms. The establishment of commonly agreed terms for infant feeding practices has proved invaluable in coordinating research and policy formation, and in reducing misunderstanding between the actors in the issue. For example, to agree on the exact difference between 'attachment' and 'positioning' (and other terms) has enhanced breastfeeding support training. As the focus on complementary feeding becomes stronger, a common clearer vocabulary would aid discussion.

Clarity is essential for any information campaign. The great strength of the campaigns against the unethical marketing of breastmilk substitutes has been that breastfeeding is unequalled. The evidence for this statement is so powerful that this concept can be easily explained and justified. Matters are not so straightforward with complementary foods.

For example, a 2006 Philippines law (on the implementation of their Code of Marketing of Breastmilk Substitutes) recommends that babies be fed with 'fresh, natural and indigenous food'.[1] What do these three terms mean? They are all ambiguous. Ambiguous words can subvert a law's purpose. For example, the Guatemalan Code of Marketing of Breastmilk Substitutes Law defined complementary foods (in Spanish) as "*todo alimento, manufacturado o preparado localmente como complemento de la leche materno*". Most people would understand and translate this as "*all foods, whether manufactured (ie by a commercial company) or prepared locally (ie in the home or local community) as a complement to breastmilk*". The transnational baby food company Gerber challenged the law because Gerber did not want to remove the baby face picture from its baby food labels. The company won its case because their lawyer argued that the law only applied to "*foods manufactured or prepared locally*". Gerber products were imported.[2] Careless drafting made Guatemalans vulnerable to the predatory skills of an external vested interest.

Let us start with the word 'fresh'. It could merely mean 'not rotten' or it could mean 'unprocessed'. It might mean leaves and fruits picked just before consumption, a fish or animal captured alive a few minutes before preparation. But many labels on jars of baby foods state: "*made with fresh ingredients*". I can guess that the drafters of the Philippines law intended to mean the preparation of unpackaged foodstuffs gathered from home-grown sources or bought in local markets. Not all market food is fresh. In some regions it is customary to buy a live chicken or fish and kill it just before or during the cooking. In other societies, including my own, it is culturally unacceptable and officially illegal to sell and buy live animals (except for molluscs and shellfish) for immediate consumption. Vegetables and fruits may be sold a few hours after gathering but, if transported in the hot sun, their vitamin levels are reduced. How food is harvested, covered, packed and displayed is important for infants and young children because of the risk of pathogenic contamination and nutrient decay. We value fresh fruit and vegetables yet a toddler may get more vitamins from frozen peas than if he is fed peas left on a sunny market stall all day. Specially designed machines can harvest vegetables in record time. Controlled blanching and freezing in factories near the fields can inactivate the intrinsic enzymes which cause deterioration within the produce, and thus conserve vitamins.

Many foodstuffs are improved by not being 'fresh' but by being processed. Cassava is poisonous unless steeped and pounded. As described in chapter 14, processes such as the liming of maize flour or the fermentation of cereals, milks and vegetables can enhance nutrient content, digestibility and storage safety. Many cheeses improve with age and retain their nutritional value. Also, drying, salting and pickling can be safer for storage in hot climates where refrigeration is absent or unreliable. Dried or salted fish was a staple food for centuries, especially in regions (eg Iceland) where neither grain nor fruit could be cultivated.[3] Highly salted food is not good for infants and young children and should be avoided. However, many traditional preserved foods are nutritionally valuable and introducing them to the young child may establish diverse long-term eating habits.

The term 'natural' is fraught with even more problems. 'Natural' does not always equate with 'good'. My description above of prehistoric diets has not included a history of how humans learned to recognise poisonous products. In the same way that people noticed positive effects of certain foods on health, strength or healing, trial and error meant that human groups had to deduce from illness or death of an individual that a certain berry, mushroom or part of an animal was harmful.* There are many examples of 'natural' foods which do harm. In 2001 in the Solomon Islands an entire family became seriously ill and several members died, including an exclusively breastfed baby, after the family had feasted on a hawksbill turtle.** It had probably eaten

---

* For example polar bear liver is poisonous to humans because of its high levels of vitamin A. Someone had to die from eating the liver for this to be known.

** Personal communication: Dr Robert Challen who was working in the Solomon Islands in 2001. Hawksbill turtles are part of the traditional diet of

toxic algae 'blooms' which occur periodically at sea. Wild foods have many health advantages but a good food can change to bad. For example, if quails (small game birds) eat the poisonous plant hemlock* they do not suffer, but a human who eats that quail is likely to die.

Vegetables and fruits can contain negative traits. Some are high in oxalic acid which, when cooked and consumed, binds with certain minerals (eg calcium) making them unavailable to the body. Spinach is high in oxalic acid. The spinach-promoting message in the 20th-century US cartoon films about 'Popeye the sailor man', was based on an arithmetical error about the iron content of spinach by public health scientists. Spinach is not particularly good for babies (and how clever they are to reject it), though a little in a diverse diet should not matter.

Lathyrism is a form of poisoning caused by eating too much of a particular legume.** In cassava-eating communities there are sporadic outbreaks of tropical paralysis (tropical ataxia) caused by the cyanide in cassava. A 1981 outbreak in Northern Mozambique was attributed to the selection of a more drought-resistant cassava variety containing higher levels of cyanide. Other food shortages led to shortened processing time so that the cyanide was not fully leached out. The selection of the different cassava occurred by exchange between subsistence farmers and had nothing to do with any company marketing or government initiative.

Iodine deficiency is 'natural' and widespread, with 2.2 billion people at risk and rates varying depending on the region.[4] Sustained and routine iodine fortification of foods or salt is the most effective way to combat it. This has to be done through

---

Pacific Islanders. These turtles are omnivorous but favour certain sponges which are toxic to other animals. They also like areas of brown algae. Either of these factors could have transferred toxins to the consumers.

* Hemlock (*Conium maculatum*) is a tall umbelliferous plant. The Greek philosopher Socrates (469BCE-399BCE) was made to drink a potion of hemlock as a form of execution.

** Botanical name: *Lathyrus sativus*; in English it is called the lathyrus pea.

factory processing. It is difficult and expensive to persuade people to eat seafoods and seaweed when they are unaccustomed to them and live far from the sea. Some common 'natural and healthy' vegetables, such as brassicas, contain goitrogens which inhibit the utilisation of iodine. These may be irrelevant if you have seafood in your diet but may be a risk if you do not. Iodine-fortified food is not 'natural' but a child whose mother is iodine deficient is likely to be less intelligent or to be born with cretinism. In this case an artificially fortified product is welcome.

'Indigenous' is a problematic term.[5*] It means innate or native to a locality. If we in Europe only ate indigenous foods, we would forego potatoes, rice, tomatoes, maize, coffee, tea, chocolate, spices, turkeys and many other foods. As mentioned in chapter 9, the introduction of foods across the world can increase diversity of eating. There are several regions of the world where a child fed only on fresh, natural and indigenous foods could become malnourished.

All terms have their problems. 'Local or locally available food' is often used. For many urban families (50% of the world's population) cola drinks and mass-produced 'fast food' are locally available foods. Are these good for infants and young children? It is not for me to decide which terms are best but to urge a considered process to achieve clarity, and to warn against making generalised statements which may lead to misunderstanding and harm infant health and development. The context is everything.

---

* The definition of 'indigenous' can be extrapolated from ecological theories which judge that any plant (or animal) introduced after 1500 CE is 'non-indigenous'. Therefore outside the Americas the potato and the tomato are non-indigenous plants. See footnote on page 42.

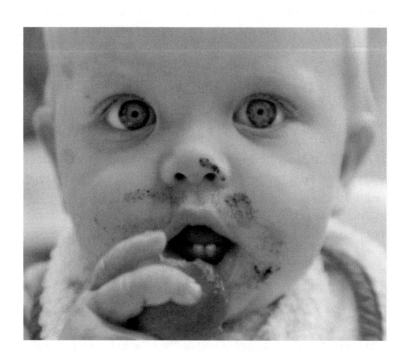

19

IS A 'LOCAL' DIET POSSIBLE AND GOOD ENOUGH FOR INFANTS AND YOUNG CHILDREN?

Some nutritionists have claimed that it is impossible to feed a child adequate nutrients without fortified industrialised products.

Poverty causes undernutrition. The children's charity Save the Children states that cash is the missing ingredient to tackle hunger. In Ethiopia the Productive Safety Nets Programme provides 7.2 million people with 30 Birr ($3.50) per head per month for seven months during the lean season. More than 70% of this cash is spent on food, and mothers report that they can then feed their children with a greater variety of food.[1]

When families have sufficient income, high education levels, and access to unbiased and accurate information they are capable of feeding their children adequately with a diet based on local foods. The Fife Diet (see box on following page) provides a contemporary European example.

We have to return to Sen's theory of entitlement (page 13). Most financially secure families could feed their children well from family foods if, like the Small family in Fife, they had access to unbiased information and the confidence to withstand marketing messages. Their money and inclusion in the social infrastructure entitles them to make rational decisions. The Fife Diet showed that a predominantly local diet with a small quantity of imported ingredients, some of which were industrially processed (eg soya sauce), could keep a whole family well nourished. This community challenged a national culture of industrialised food provision and promotion. The following section shows how national policies influence eating practices.

THE FIFE DIET

In Fife, Scotland, one family, Mike and Karen Small and their children, changed their eating patterns for environmental and ethical reasons (to reduce food miles) and committed themselves to live on locally grown foods (The Fife Diet). Their son Sorley was nearly three years old, and breastfed baby, Alex, five months old when they embarked on this project. Scotland lacks sunshine and the growing season is short but produce suited to the climate is grown. The family lived on local potatoes, other root and leafy vegetables, meat, fish, eggs, butter and seasonal fruits. Karen abandoned her former vegetarianism because she had relied on so many imported foods. The few imported foods they decided to retain were: coffee, tea, chocolate, spices, lemons, peanut butter and soya sauce. Doubters claimed that the Fife diet was nutritionally irresponsible and might impair the health of their children. In fact the family consume nutritious and delicious food and the children are thriving. Their food preparation time doubled but their costs almost halved.[*]

The Smalls no longer eat commercially manufactured snacks, such as biscuits. They do not have scurvy or any other nutrient deficiencies. An example list of a week's meals indicates a diverse and balanced diet that can meet all their children's needs.

The project originally started with 14 people and now has 600 participants. They are currently exploring the possibility of cultivating quinoa in their area.[2]

---

[*] The Small family's weekly food bill went down from around £100.00 to between £50.00 and £60.00. UK median weekly wage at the time of reporting was £479.00. At that time it was estimated that a healthy diet and minimum basket of necessities for a family of four cost £67.00 a week. The Smalls were able to access local fresh food; in poor urban areas this may not be possible.

20

A LESSON FROM HISTORY: THE EXAMPLE OF WARTIME UK

In 1937, two years before the onset of the Second World War, a study revealed that out of a population of 41 million people in the UK, 32 million had some nutritional deficiencies and four and a half million were deficient in every nutrient. Only a wealthy minority consumed sufficient to meet their basic dietary requirements. Nutritional status was strongly related to income.[1] There is a parallel situation in many developing countries today.

At the outbreak of war, a comprehensive food policy was devised and led by The Ministry of Food (MOF). Much thought and planning went into the policy.[2] The goal was to protect the population from the effects of food shortages. Agricultural policy, food quality, availability and distribution were centrally coordinated by the MOF. Rationing, devised to maximise nutritional advantage, provided equal food distribution for all. Despite food shortages and other wartime deprivations, the results of this policy led to remarkable improvements in mother and child health. Infant, neonatal and maternal mortality and stillbirths reached their lowest levels in British history. Incidence of iron-deficiency anaemia and dental caries declined and the growth of schoolchildren improved. Tuberculosis control also improved.*

There was nationwide public health and nutrition education through mass media. MOF advertisements such as *'Welcome little stranger'* gave advice on eating in pregnancy and *'Don't let Dad get all the meat'* directed household food distribution. Public awareness of the relationship between food and health grew. This was achieved through clearly disseminated knowledge,

---

* NB: These improvements predated the formation of the National Health Service and also the use of antibiotics.

use of locally available foods and respect for family skills, and carried out without food industry pressures. It was assumed that complementary feeding would be derived from family foods. Successful media messages urged that young children should take priority in the family distribution of the more nutritious foods. The same communications explained which foods were the most nutritious. Breastfeeding was the norm but provision of state-supplied breastmilk substitutes was introduced. This was because adverse 20th century practices (eg restricted breastfeeding) meant that some women 'could not breastfeed'.*

Key factors in this success were government control of food supplies and the inclusion of the scientific experts in Ministry decision making. Another aspect was that increased numbers of women joined all levels of the labour force and contributed to decision-making processes. This was due to the absence of men and not because of any drive for gender equality.

So remarkable were these achievements that in 1947 the American Public Health Association presented The Lasker Group Award to "*The British Ministries of Food and Health for the unprecedented program of food distribution in Great Britain, with resulting improvement in the health of the people*". [3]

This British experience has been consigned to history and is often viewed with mere sentiment but its lessons are relevant to the 21st century. The fact that a simple system transformed child nutrition and health for the better in adverse circumstances, within a very short period of time, provides an evidence-based model for contemporary societies struggling to improve mother and child nutrition (see Appendix III).

---

* Restricting breastfeeding through routines was promoted by the medical profession so 'insufficient milk' did occur. *Sevrage* between six and nine months was the norm but, depending on the region, poorer women breastfed for longer. State-manufactured 'National Dried Milk' was provided for children up to two years of age. It was not promoted or on sale in shops but leaflets instructed application to The Food Office or Welfare Centre. Branded breastmilk substitutes were available and promoted but were too expensive for the mass of the people.

A CONTEMPORARY LESSON: US SPECIAL SUPPLEMENTAL PROGRAMME FOR WOMEN, INFANTS AND CHILDREN (WIC)

The US Special Supplemental Nutrition Programme for Women, Infants and Children (WIC) was authorised by the 1966 US Child Nutrition Act. It was launched in 1974 and during that year 88,000 people participated. By 2008 average monthly participation was 8.2 million. WIC was and is targeted to poor women, infants and children to improve their nutrition and health, and provides food directly to recipients. WIC cannot serve all eligible people and uses a priority system to select those at most nutrition risk.[1]

Being a WIC recipient is a sign of poverty and carries some stigma. Food provision may disempower mothers because it slants and restricts their food decisions. The WIC programme provides breastmilk substitutes and specific foods or vouchers. It does not appear to have significantly improved nutritional awareness and child feeding skills. It has probably had a negative effect on breastfeeding.

Poor mothers are more likely to be WIC participants and have children who are less healthy. Within the USA there is a correlation between income inequality and infant mortality rates (IMR). For example, Louisiana, with wide income differentials, has more than double the IMR of Alaska, one of the most equal states.[2] Though it may have ameliorated the ill effects of other economic and social problems, one cannot present WIC as a model for the development of beneficial infant and young child feeding policies. US income differentials are the widest of any industrialised country. In 2009 the USA ranked 43rd in world IMR data.[3]

These comments are not intended to deprecate the work

of those who strive to make the WIC programme effective in protecting health and nutrition. In recent years there have been WIC breastfeeding programmes and other nutrition education inputs and changes to the content of the food package are ongoing.[4] It is probable that in the early days WIC prevented undernutrition. Nevertheless, the fact that in the 21st century a sophisticated, industrialised country has to provide foods for such a substantial proportion of mothers, infants and children – and commit such a large amount of public expenditure to do this – is a gloomy model for developing nations (see Appendix IV).

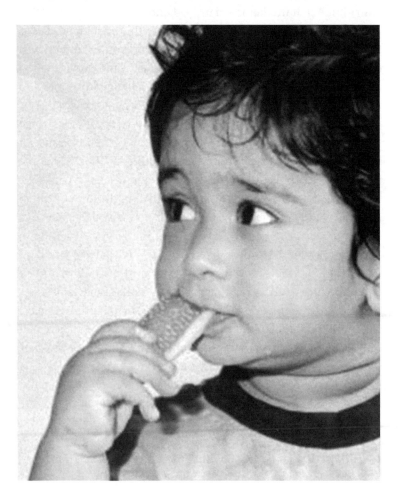

22

THE MAJORITY WORLD

To return to my experience in Mozambique: despite war, economic collapse and entrenched poverty, some older infants and young children did very well. The doctor with whom I worked did some rapid research. We found that the children who thrived had family in both the city and the countryside. Food was rarely available on the open market* and, in the capital city Maputo, citizens depended on local government distribution of a monthly ration of staple cereal (maize meal or rice), coconut oil and sugar. Vegetables, fruit, eggs, meat and fish were available only sporadically and were snapped up by people with connections. We discovered that if a child's family had entitlement to the monthly ration and also produced food in the countryside, then that child was less likely to become undernourished.

One approach to infant and young child feeding has been to address specific nutrient deficiencies. Vitamin A, zinc, iodine and iron deficiencies contribute most to infant and young child mortality.[1] They are associated with the conditions of poverty, the region a child lives in and food insecurity. Some specific programmes of technical intervention have proved useful. Iodine deficiency declines with economic development because dietary diversification increases when people can buy imported food produced in iodine-rich regions. However, many people still subsist on locally produced food. If they live in an iodine-deficient region they and their children are at risk. In this case routine fortification (eg through iodised salt) can be a beneficial strategy.**

---

* There was no functioning market. The only food products on open sale were tea, garlic, leaves and occasionally tomatoes. Most trading was through a small black market and a tiny, hard-currency shop.

** For example: when Papua New Guinea introduced legislation banning the import or trade of non-iodised salt, the prevalence of goitres and cretinism

This requires coordinated action at national and international level. Such initiatives have worked well and are examples of an industrialised process providing a nutritional benefit.[2]

But the delivery of synthetic nutrients through programming does not always bring such beneficial results. During the late 20th century, programmes to deliver synthetic vitamin A doses to newborns were hailed as a way to reduce levels of infant infection and death. However, a 2009 review of neonatal vitamin A supplementation found no reduced risk of common morbidities (diarrhoea and others), admission to hospital or mortality. Moreover there was an increased risk of acute respiratory infection. The authors conclude that there is no justification for such supplementation.[3] A costly and 'top-down' system has failed to achieve its goals.

These researchers also uncovered another uncomfortable fact: in their scrutiny of these studies, they could not find much data on maternal night blindness prevalence and low birth weights. Night blindness indicates vitamin A deficiency and is more common during pregnancy because mothers' vitamin A requirements increase. In some poor societies it is so common that it is considered a normal sign in pregnancy. Poor nutrition in pregnancy is a leading cause of low birth weight in the majority world. Both conditions reveal the state of women's nutrition. The fact that so many studies omitted to gather data about these conditions speaks loudly about the status of women and their human rights.[4*]

It is mostly women, and especially mothers, who do the complementary feeding. If a mother's own nutrition is neglected she is more likely to have a low birth weight baby whose mortality risk is greater. Such babies can have more difficulties breastfeeding and, without skilled assistance, there is more pressure to introduce complementary foods too early, which increases the

---

dropped significantly.

* Since I first wrote this, there has been investigation into women's night blindness and the effects of vitamin A supplementation. The results showed no benefit.

risk of illness and death. More importantly, an undernourished mother whose vision is impaired is less likely to be able to prepare complementary foods hygienically or feed a baby when light is poor. Moreover, she needs to be healthy to attend to her child's needs.

Breastfeeding is biologically robust; even a weak mother can carry on suckling when she is ill, but complementary feeding takes initiative, activity and energy. A woman has to obtain sufficient food, fetch water and buy soap to do all the preparation hygienically; she must contrive to allocate the most nutritious morsels for her child, often in competition with other family members. She may deprive herself of food to do this. This is all on top of her normal work burden, which can be overwhelming even when she is healthy. If she is herself nutrient deficient then it may be impossible. If she delegates the complementary feeding to other family members, can she ensure their hygiene skills or devotion to the baby? Might hungry siblings be tempted to eat the baby's portion? Good complementary feeding cannot happen if women's right to nutrition is ignored.

There is another aspect to the link between the nutrition and health of mothers and their children. A baby in the womb of a nutritionally deprived mother will be programmed to withstand the harsh environment of food scarcity. If that baby is fed a diet that is too energy dense (ie too high in calories) he may be more vulnerable to long-term diseases such as diabetes.[5] Genetic research has shown that there are physiological, intergenerational effects that may be traced back even to grandparents. As one public health expert said: *"We used to say, you are what you eat; now we know, you are what your mother ate."*[6] This means a woman's lifelong nutrition from her own birth, not merely a good diet during pregnancy. Transforming the nutrition of girls and women is essential for babies to be born healthy. Just as with delayed umbilical cord clamping and exclusive breastfeeding, what goes before complementary feeding is as important as the nature of the feeding itself.

I do not want to suggest that all supplementation programmes are wrong. Some nutrient supplementation for older babies and young children may remain a necessity as long as food insecurity is neglected. The provision of synthetic nutrients can provide a vital bridge for survival while society resolves its food systems and poverty. However, such interventions should always be under review. For example, routine iron supplementation of pregnant women is a good public health strategy while iron-deficiency anaemia prevalence is high. When overall nutrition improves, the risks outweigh the benefits. Then, only women with diagnosed iron-deficiency anaemia should be supplemented.

It seems in the 21st century that nutrient supplementation initiatives do not build withdrawal into their implementation plans. For example, vitamin A supplementation programmes did not appear to include measures for closure. Is it assumed that poor sanitation and inadequate diets will last forever? The late-20th-century political drive for public-private partnerships could be interpreted as the state handing over responsibility for nutrition to the profit-making sector, while side-stepping the central role of family skills and household self-sufficiency. For example, the Global Alliance for Improved Nutrition (GAIN) was launched in 2002 as *"an alliance of international public, private and civic organisations committed to improving health, cognitive development and productivity in developing countries through the elimination of vitamin and mineral deficiencies – especially deficiencies of vitamin A, folic acid and iron"*. The main aim of this *"alliance of public and private sector partners"* was to *"leverage cost-effective food fortification initiatives"* to achieve this goal.[7]

A 2008 WHO/UNICEF report states that *"there are not enough well-documented, large scale programmes that have successfully improved feeding practices in children 6-23 months of age and resulted in improved outcomes"*.[8] A systematic review of interventions concludes that there is no universal best package and that educational approaches can be effective, especially when combined with home fortification or provision of fortified foods. Any provision of food must be modest to avoid displacement of breastmilk.[9] This report also concludes that context is crucial.

The so-called 'developing world' is not developing. Within most international nutrition and health documents there is an intrinsic and almost fatalistic 'them and us' stance as though there are two separate planets occupied by the rich and the poor. There are however well-documented programmes of national child health improvements in regions that had experienced high rates of child undernutrition in the past, such as Kerala State in India, Cuba and parts of Europe.

Lessons can be learned from the two systems designed to protect mother and child nutrition, described in the sections on the UK during the Second World War and the WIC programme in the USA. (3.3 and 3.4). Both included the goal of protecting and improving infant and young child nutrition. The former succeeded in a remarkably short period of time. The latter may have inadvertently contributed to an entrenched culture of adverse infant and young child eating practices within an underclass.

International agencies attempt to tackle child nutrition issues with guidance constrained by political pressures. The Global Strategy for Infant and Young Child Feeding (GSIYCF) emphasises the need for accurate information and skilled support from the family, community and healthcare system. It calls for diversified approaches and suggests home- and community-based technologies to enhance nutrient density, bioavailability and the micronutrient content of local foods. It also states that, *"Industrially processed complementary foods also provide an option for some mothers who have the means to buy them and the knowledge and facilities to prepare them safely."* [10]

There is a risk contained within this information. If elite mothers in any community buy and use industrially processed complementary foods this creates a two-tier food system and motivates poor mothers to buy such foods. The marketing of these foods exploits parental aspirations, exaggerates the nutritional benefits of the foods and undermines impartial messages about locally available foods. Such marketing is usually designed to normalise their use and imply that they are essential.

The current practice of setting up local community

manufacture of nutritionally adequate complementary foods is seen in many quarters as the compromise answer. There are inherent dangers. If the enterprise is well run, successful and creates a functioning local demand for the product then this will inevitably attract large-scale manufacturers to buy out the enterprise and eventually dominate the local market. The fact that the giant international baby food company Danone is an active working partner within the international private-public partnership the Global Alliance for Improved Nutrition (GAIN), and that GAIN is seen by many powerful donors as the route to the conquest of infant and young child undernutrition, highlights this problem.* Is the goal to support a well-informed population to feed their children primarily within the home, from locally available foods, or to establish an international market for transnational manufacturers?

The lesson from the UK Second World War experience shows that national awareness and skills can be enhanced and supported in a very short space of time in extremely difficult circumstances and lead to real improvements in health and nutrition. The lesson from the US WIC Programme experience is that de-skilling and dependency can transfer power to the infant food manufacturers who have a vested interest in maintaining the system. The fact that such a large tranche of public subsidy could survive the era of neo-liberal economics attests to the stranglehold of a strong vested interest. What should have been a temporary solution to an economic problem of a disadvantaged minority group has become a permanent and narrow approach which lacks the capacity to address the root causes. It is possible that the GAIN initiative carries the same dangers.

---

*   This may have changed by the time this book is in print. Currently Danone is exceeded only by Nestlé as a dominator of the world baby food market.

KEY POINTS FROM PART THREE

- The words and terms used in the discussion of complementary feeding and foods can cause confusion and the establishment of agreed terms would be helpful.

- Not all industrially processed foods are bad and not all 'natural' foods are good.

- Poverty is the major cause of child undernutrition and malnutrition.

- Context is everything.

- The British nutrition and food policy and experience during the Second World War (1939-45) provides an example of a successful food and nutrition strategy.

- The US WIC policy and experience provides an example of how nutrition support can be costly and lead to unforeseen negative consequences.

- Programmes to tackle specific nutrient deficiencies can be successful.

- Adequate complementary feeding depends on food security.

- The fulfilment and respect for women's right to adequate nutrition is essential for adequate complementary feeding.

- There are intergenerational influences on nutrition which highlight the fact that the nutrition of infants and young children should not be addressed separately from that of women.

- Current global public-private initiatives damage and disempower families.

- Complacency about global differentials restricts progress.

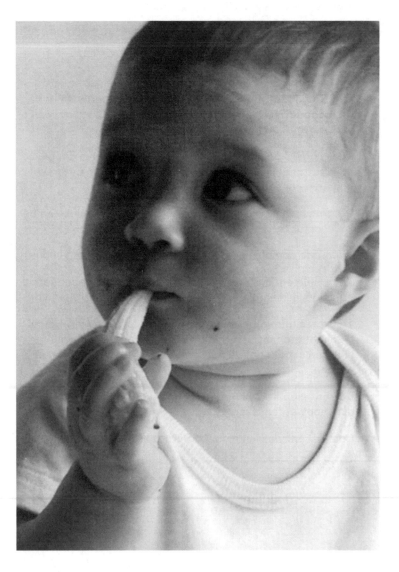

AFTERWORD: HEALTH FOR ALL?

In 1978 the Alma Ata International Conference on Primary Health Care took place and its Declaration was adopted as the policy model for global health.[1] Its strapline was *"Health for All by the Year 2000"*. A short booklet published by IBFAN (International Baby Food Action Network) in 2008 asks a question in its title: "*Whatever happened to Health for All?*"[2] The author, Lida Lhotska, challenges the amnesia about the key importance of primary health care and the implementation of global policies that could prevent ill health. Her focus is on the experience of campaigns on breastfeeding and the regulation of marketing of breastmilk substitutes, but the text applies just as well to the solid foods we give our children. Such experts as Dr Lhotska have always agreed that some industrially processed foods may be necessary and useful in certain circumstances, but she and her colleagues have shown through their work that regulation of marketing is essential. The situation regarding complementary feeding is exactly the same as that for breastmilk substitutes. Parents and carers pour money into the coffers of companies to buy food for their children that is at best unnecessary and at worst harmful. I am not talking about disaster situations here but at the level of ordinary family life in both rich and poor countries.

Governments and international health agencies appear impotent to control the actions of transnational companies; documents written by international health agencies tend to sidestep the problem and ignore 'the elephant in the room' of misleading marketing information and undue influence on government policies. For example, many of those who contributed to scientific meetings or policy-making sessions towards the end of the 20th century were aware that the public statement from the World Health Organisation (WHO) – that complementary foods were unnecessary or even harmful before six months – was delayed because of pressure from the baby food industry.

In the foreword to *"Whatever happened to Health for All?"* there is reference to price rises of staple foods and food riots: it continues *"One by one, these crises have demonstrated the weakness of market based solutions and have underscored the urgency of providing adequate protection to the world's peoples to safeguard their health, safety and livelihoods. Sustainable, affordable solutions already exist, but may be threatened by market forces seeking to place private profit above public health."* [3]

We know that shamefully large numbers of children in both wealthy and poverty-stricken regions suffer malnutrition: the malnutrition of excess amounts of inappropriate foods and the malnutrition of insufficient nutritious food. As adults we should feel embarrassed that so many small children are so poorly fed. We can change this situation if we want to and many people are already working to this end. Good nutrition for children harmonises with good nutrition for adults . . . and it would be good for the whole world if we worked to this end.

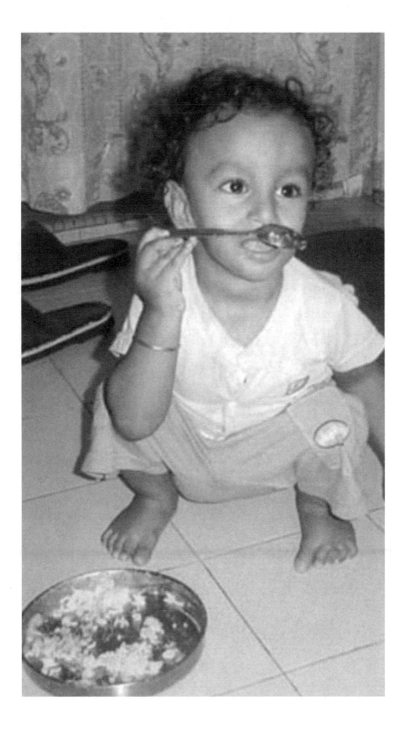

APPENDICES

Appendix I

INSECTS AND OTHER INVERTEBRATES AS FOOD

I Prevalence of consumption

Insects and other small invertebrates have always been part of the human diet. As Alan Davidson says: *"It is only in the western world, and in recent times, that it has been viewed as a strange or even revolting practice."* [1] They are used both as drought season foods and as delicacies in many countries around the world. Currently, 1,509 species of insects are eaten by 3,000 ethnic groups across 120 countries. These include caterpillars, locusts and beetles, of which 443 species are consumed.[2] Many are seasonal treats. Professor Peter Pharoah filmed 20th-century toddlers in Papua New Guinea catching insects and spiders for food.[3] Also eaten are insect products such as the papery substance making up ant and wasp nests or the golden globe of sugary liquid carried by the honey ant. Honey from bees is widely favoured.

Other small and nutrient-dense invertebrates include snails. French *'escargots'* have become elite delicacies but in the 1970s I snacked on miscellaneous cooked garden snails in a bar in central Portugal. In the open food markets of China I have eaten silk worms, scorpion and locusts, deliciously prepared and served on skewers. I have also enjoyed the dried caterpillars eaten in Southern Africa. In Northern Thailand, consumption of diverse small vertebrates and invertebrates is normal. A prestige sauce is made from a translucent, perfumed secretion extracted from the 'pimp beetle'.[4] The shock or even disgust that so often greets this information is a good example of how our emotions have a powerful influence on our eating habits.

2 Nutrition

Insects and related products can provide nutrient-dense food for older infants and young children. The hard outer casing of insects such as beetles (called chitin, the equivalent of a prawn's shell) is not digestible but in other respects most insects or their larvae are extremely nutritious. Some are rich in fats and therefore energy dense; most contain significant proportions of protein, vitamins and minerals. The high content of iron and zinc is of particular interest.[5] It may be that the inevitable inclusion of some unseen insects or their larvae in plant foods provides the vitamin B12 that is found only in animal products. If this is so then pesticides could be viewed as anti-nutrients.

Once again, the ever quotable Alan Davidson sums up the state of affairs in his recommendation of the key book on insects as food:[6] *"(Insect) consumption is hardly ever reflected in official statistics. This is partly because a single insect, although it may provide useful protein, fat and carbohydrate, furnishes only trivial amounts; partly because there are no sophisticated marketing arrangements for insects, such as would bring them within the scope of data on imports and exports; and partly, perhaps, because the class of data compilers hardly overlaps at all with the class of insect eaters."* [7]

These 'trivial amounts' of nutrients might make all the difference to a child fed on the predominantly starchy staple diet that is commonplace throughout the world.

3 Cultural attitudes

In Mozambique in 1982, owing to civil war, economic collapse and food scarcity, child malnutrition was prevalent. Ministry of Health nutritionists designed a poster urging mothers to add nutrient-dense products to the staple maize porridge fed to older infants and young children. Suggestions were meat, fish, eggs (all hard to get), ground peanuts and cashews, caterpillars and locusts. Despite the traditional use of the latter two products the Deputy Minister of Health (DMH) forbade their mention on the poster, *"because the South Africans might read them and think we are starving"*. The fact that some children were indeed starving was overridden by concerns about national identity. The DMH believed such information might make Mozambicans appear 'uncivilised'.

Many Europeans and North Americans express disgust at the idea of insect consumption yet a red colouring matter from the immature cochineal insect is widely used in foodstuffs.* It is more stable and is considered safer than synthetic red colouring matter.

In 2009, a South Korean team won the Microsoft 'Imagine Cup' top prize for a system to help people farm insect foods in famine areas. Stag beetle cookies were made in Gabon, Africa, and were eaten with pleasure.[8]

NB: Caution is needed when there is a focus on special foods for famine situations. 'Branding' foods specifically for disadvantaged groups or situations may lead to a scorn for those foods in normal circumstances.

---

* The cochineal beetle (*Dactylopius coccus*) is found on or farmed on certain cacti, harvested and processed into carmine food and cosmetic colouring. Many consumers trust its safety more than synthetic dyes.

Appendix II

A NUTRIENT EXAMPLE: IRON

I An iron-deficiency anaemia lesson

I have chosen to discuss just one nutrient to give an example of the complexities of one crucial nutrient. This does not mean other nutrients are not important.

Current textbooks state that two billion humans suffer from iron-deficiency anaemia, making this the most common nutritional deficiency syndrome. Menstruating and pregnant women are at particular risk. Iron-deficiency anaemia in infants and young children impairs their development.

One reason for the choice of iron as the example nutrient for this book is that most iron-rich food sources also supply zinc. These are the two priority nutrients not fully met by breastmilk as a child reaches the end of her first year. The timing of any actual deficiency will depend on the child's body stores of iron at birth. The small proportion of iron in breastmilk is highly bioavailable. In evolutionary terms larger amounts in breastmilk were unnecessary because our ancestors' children got the iron they needed from external sources. Cows' milk is a poor source of iron; moreover its consumption during a meal inhibits the absorption of iron in other foods. Using milk as a vehicle for iron fortification (as in follow-on milks) is illogical. I will discuss dietary inhibitors and enhancers of iron in section 4, below.

Iron deficiency and iron-deficiency anaemia are not the same thing. The human body stores iron in the bone marrow and serum. Iron is essential for many roles in our bodies, for example to form haemoglobin in red blood cells, which transport oxygen throughout the body. Free iron is highly toxic, so it is normally bound by protective proteins such as ferritin and transferrin (its job is to *transfer*), which prevent the iron from damaging the body. It is the iron in haemoglobin which makes our blood red. Iron is 'recycled' around the body. However, if iron is lost from blood loss due to injury, parasitic infection or menstrual periods, this must be replaced from sources outside the body. Without replacement through the diet, iron stores in the bone marrow and serum become depleted. As stores decline, absorption of iron into the bloodstream becomes more efficient. However, if iron stores become too low, then haemoglobin production is impaired. This is iron deficiency.

Iron-deficiency anaemia (IDA) is another matter. Countries and health agencies have differing criteria for what are acceptable haemoglobin values. Iron-deficiency anaemia occurs in an individual when haemoglobin levels fall below the 2.5 percentile of a given country's stated values, so its definition is a statistical nicety. Suppose that Country X decides that anaemia occurs when a woman has a serum ferritin (iron store) level of less than 17 micrograms per litre (ɥg/l), while nearby Country Y sets the value at 16ɥg/l. A woman from Country X with a serum ferritin level of 16.5ɥg/l could theoretically stop being anaemic simply by walking across the border to Country Y. This is not a joke and does in fact cause problems. In the late 20th century experts contested UNICEF's statements about the global prevalence of IDA because of differing assessment methods.[1]

In reality, it is the clinical assessment of an individual's signs and symptoms that is important. People vary: one woman, carrying out physical labour without feeling tired, may have a lower haemoglobin value than another woman, who does no hard work but is breathless and exhausted. This condition can become so severe that oxygen delivery to the vital organs is impaired. Many women in developing countries have died of heart failure during their prime years because of such levels of IDA. If a child is growing well and full of energy one can be relaxed about his iron status; if he is listless, tired and without appetite, one should be concerned. Iron-deficiency anaemia is associated with impairment of cognitive development in children as well as other developmental problems.

The second important point is that iron can be dangerous. Too much iron damages the vital organs. Groups who brew beer in iron pots, drink excessive amounts of red wine or self-medicate with over-the-counter iron tablets are all at risk. Iron supplementation could be fatal for certain populations with genetic traits that make absorption of dietary iron too efficient, leading to iron overload. It can also prove fatal if given too early during the rehabilitation of severely malnourished children, even though they are usually iron deficient.

Pathogens thrive in the presence of iron. One of the many roles of the breastmilk protein, lactoferrin is to bind with iron so that it does not become available to pathogens in the baby's gut. About 50 to 70% of the small quantity of iron in breastmilk is absorbed. In contrast only about 12% of the larger quantities of iron in iron-fortified infant formula is absorbed. This can be a risk to a newborn's immature kidneys, which may be unable to excrete the excess iron in these artificial feeds.

2 Iron-deficiency anaemia is a global health problem

Despite the controversies of definitions and diagnoses, we can confidently state that iron-deficiency anaemia is a major global public health problem. Iron requirements are high in infants after about six months (depending on their birth stores, see below), in young children, and in menstruating and pregnant women. Lactational amenorrhoea provides some protection from IDA for lactating women. The levels of iron in breastmilk are remarkably consistent and are not influenced by a mother's diet or her iron stores.

Evidence about early human diets indicates that babies and toddlers met their iron needs. It must therefore be asked why so many modern children suffer IDA. During the 20th century some nutritionists stated that no mother could provide enough iron in her child's diet. Some argued that a small child would need to eat a kilo of liver a day to meet her needs and therefore that synthetic fortification of infant foods (inevitably industrially produced) was the only answer. In a discussion with a nutritionist colleague who argued for this policy I asked this question: *"If you believe that no child can derive sufficient iron from food, are you suggesting that Socrates, Jesus, Mohammed, Galileo, Einstein, Marie Curie and others with great talent and wisdom, would all have had better brains if they had eaten iron-fortified cereals?"* To my astonishment he replied, *"Yes"*. Some nutritionists seem to forget that one can only judge the strength of theories by results. If millions of human beings have grown up to be strong, healthy and intelligent without synthetically fortified foods then these calculations must be wrong.

There are evidently other routes to satisfactory iron status. In the 1980s, scientist Professor Peter Hartmann described an Australian child exclusively breastfed at 15 months. A British Professor of Nutrition asked Peter if he had looked at this child's iron status. *"No"* replied Peter *"I couldn't catch him."* [2] Clearly there are many confounding factors as to why some children have IDA and others do not. Living in a developing country or being poor in a rich one are both key risk factors. Nevertheless it is important to understand some some basic facts about iron deficiency anaemia.

3 Does good complementary feeding start before birth? A mother's iron status plus early cord clamping

The Australian child mentioned above thrived on exclusive breastfeeding long after he was supposed to. It is likely that he was born with optimal iron stores; that his mother was well nourished, ate a diet rich in meat and fish, and therefore maintained good iron status throughout her pregnancy. If her haemoglobin during pregnancy had fallen below Australian IDA levels she would have received iron and folate supplementation. Iron deficiency does not occur because of insufficient dietary iron alone. Iron-deficiency anaemia is associated with poverty, an impoverished diet and other nutrient deficiencies.

Well-nourished mothers produce babies who are born with a store of iron which will last them well into the second half-year of life. From this we can conclude that respecting women's human rights to economic justice and to food might be a more effective strategy for reducing IDA in infants and young children than providing iron-enriched foods for infants.

Many common birth practices worldwide are regrettable. In too many regions it is still normal for women to give birth on their backs and suffer unnecessary and/or harmful interventions such as shaving, episiotomy, routine use of drugs and non-essential caesarean sections. These practices harm women, undermine exclusive breastfeeding and sabotage infant iron status.

Early cord clamping is the norm in hospitals all over the world in both rich and poor settings. It is only necessary in a minority of situations, where the baby's or mother's life is at stake. Birth attendants should wait at least two minutes, or until the cord stops pulsating, before clamping. This allows a significant transfer of blood from the placenta to the baby and makes a difference to babies' long-term iron stores, especially those born to mothers with low iron levels themselves.[3]

In some industrialised countries, there have been proposals that cord blood should be routinely harvested to gather stem cells, in case that individual needs them in later life. Such harvesting deprives a baby of her rightful blood and reduces her iron stores; 100ml of blood from a newborn is equivalent to taking over a litre from an adult.[4] When breastfeeding mothers are harassed and made anxious about their babies' haemoglobin levels, the question they should ask is, *"Who deprived my baby of her placental blood transfer?"*

An effective global campaign against early umbilical cord cutting might lead to a decline in IDA in infants. It would require two minutes per birth of hospital staff time. Birth attendants could find another useful ritual to perform (maybe collecting their breath) during those two minutes. Such a pause would have the added benefit of facilitating unhurried postnatal skin-to-skin contact between a mother and her baby, which is crucial for successful breastfeeding.

4 Iron bioavailaility: inhibitors and enhancers

The quantity of iron in the diet is less important than its bioavailability. Dietary iron comes in two forms: flesh foods such as meat, fish and molluscs contain haem iron; plant foods contain non-haem iron. Haem iron is more bioavailable than non-haem iron. This does not mean that a predominantly plant food diet is iron deficient but that dietary practices influence bioavailability. A plant-food-based diet has health advantages for the whole family, but the proportion of animal foods should be geared towards the older infant and young child. In many societies, adults, particularly men, appropriate the animal products[5] and children get too few. Many men in industrialised societies would benefit from a reduction in animal food consumption and most small children, especially in poor societies, would benefit from an increase. The British Second World War poster *'Don't let Dad get all the meat'* could usefully be an international slogan.

4.1 Iron inhibitors

a) Phenolic compounds are substances in plants that protect them from pests. They bind with iron and thus reduce absorption. They are plentiful in many vegetables, such as spinach, herbs, such as oregano, and some spices. They are especially high in tea, coffee and cocoa, so drinking these with food significantly reduces absorption of iron in a meal. In several regions (such as Central Asia) tea* with

---

* I am referring to Indian or China tea from the *Camellia sinensis* plant not herbal teas. NB: All such beverages are to be discouraged for infants as they interfere with exclusive breastfeeding and are unnecessary. Though research is lacking, some herbal teas may have harmful effects.

sugar is given to babies from the earliest weeks and is drunk throughout childhood. Sweetened black coffee is given to children from about nine months in Guatemala. As well as replacing breastmilk with a nutrient-poor fluid, coffee and tea can reduce iron absorption from the meal by as much as 40% (coffee) to 60% (tea).

b) Calcium reduces iron absorption. A glass of milk with a meal may reduce iron absorption by as much as 50%. Epidemiological evidence shows an association between milk intake and iron deficiency.

c) Phytates in cereals strongly inhibit iron absorption. Wholegrain cereals have higher levels of phytates than refined cereals; oats are particularly effective iron inhibitors.

d) Fibre reduces iron absorption.

e) Soy protein reduces iron absorption.

f) Prolonged cooking of meat at high temperatures reduces the bioavailability of iron.

NB: For all those who are not at risk of iron deficiency (eg men and post-menopausal women), iron-binding mechanisms may have a health advantage by protecting against iron overload.

4.2 Iron enhancers

a) The most potent iron enhancer is vitamin C. There is a wonderful synergy through eating a mixed meal. Vitamin C in fruit and vegetables enhances the absorption of iron from all other foods. Adding a small amount of meat, fish or seafood to a meal enhances absorption of non-haem iron of plant foods. Thus a few chopped fresh herbs (such as coriander, parsley or basil) or a squeeze of lemon or lime (or any fruit) on the food makes more iron available. Citric acid itself enhances iron absorption. These practices not only enhance nutrition but accustom the infant and young child to healthy eating practices for a lifetime. Almost all traditional diets have food customs which appear ritualistic but in fact enhance iron absorption. Ironically, people often omit the squeeze of lemon, the chopped herbs, or the inclusion of the animal foods when they feed the infant or young child.

b) Fermentation processes, especially of cereals, favour iron absorption.

c) Iron from the soil can be present in significant quantities on the surface of the food and may have nutritional importance. Cooking in iron pots also contributes iron to the diet.[6]

4.3 Iron fortification

If a population has eating practices that limit iron then it is only ethical to endorse iron fortification of foods. The question is whether these should be general foods, such as bread flour, or foods manufactured for babies. Sprinkles or pills of multi-vitamins and iron are another option. The issues of affordability and dependency on commercial products must be considered, as must the risk of accidental overdose.

Appendix III

ADDITIONAL INFORMATION ON THE BRITISH 'FOOD FOR VICTORY' CAMPAIGN

I Rations and rules

In 1942, a typical week's ration for an adult in the UK was 150g of bacon and cheese, six pence (£0.025) worth of meat (<500g depending on the type and cut of meat), 100g of fat, one egg, 1.2 to 1.8 litres of milk, 225g of sugar and 50g of tea. Hoarding food was a punishable offence. Wild game meats or home-reared chickens and rabbits were not rationed. Vegetable growing was strongly supported and by 1943 over a million tons of vegetables were being produced in home gardens and allotments.* Fish was not rationed but availability was haphazard. All bread flour was of higher extraction (ie less refined) and fortified with iron, vitamins and calcium. People were encouraged to forage for wild foods such as rose hips (a key source of vitamin C for children), mushrooms, berries and wild leaves. There was some black marketeering and the rich could afford occasional luxury products when available, but for the first time in British history the poorest citizens had nutritious food security. Research showed that the nation had never been so healthy. Sugar imports fell to half their pre-war levels, sweets were rationed and dental caries decreased. By 1944, expectant mothers and children were consuming more eggs and milk per head than before the war.

A recent BBC TV series, where two people live on the food of a particular historical era for one week and then measure the

---

*   Allotments are small plots of land in towns allocated for growing family food. It is still a legal requirement for local councils to provide them. I have had one for over 30 years.

physiological effects, found that the Second World War (WW2) diet made them healthier than any other diet in history.[1]

2 The Welfare Foods Scheme for women and children

The health of women, infants and children improved dramatically throughout the war. Awareness of their priority needs spread. In 1944 the maternal mortality rate was half 1938 levels. Introduced in 1941, the Welfare Foods scheme entitled pregnant women, babies and children to special or extra foods, and extra free or cheaper milk, meat, eggs and fruit. Orange juice and rose hip syrup were provided at affordable prices. Cod liver oil imported from Iceland was provided free to pregnant and breastfeeding women, children under five and adults over forty. Vitamin pills were distributed. By 1942, after an initial rise, infant mortality had fallen below pre-war levels.

3 Leaders of the programme

The food industry did not have undue influence on the policy, but had to fulfil obligations such as fortification of bread flour or vitamin D enrichment of margarine. The policy was devised by respected scientists, including Sir Jack Drummond, Sir Wilson Jameson, Sir John Boyd Orr, nutritionists Robert McCance and Elsie Widdowson, who worked closely with the government. The Minister of Food, Lord Woolton, became so famous that a vegetable pie was named after him. The healthy babies in propaganda photographs were called 'Lord Woolton's babies'.

4 Personal experience

Though born after WW2, I am a beneficiary of that system. My mother, raised on a poor diet and with no nutritional knowledge, benefited from the focus on pregnant women and infants. She bore four healthy children and fed them on the wartime diet. In contrast to pre-war culture, prioritising the child's diet in the household became normal. As a child, I learned from my mother that potatoes should be plunged into boiling water (not cold) to conserve their vitamin C; that sodium bicarbonate must not be added to the cooking of green vegetables (an old British custom to enhance the green colour) because it destroyed B vitamins; that watercress was rich in minerals and vitamins. She learned all this and how to be a thrifty and imaginative cook from wartime propaganda. As one author wrote, *"Never before have the British people been so wisely fed or British women so sensibly interested in cooking."*[2]

5 Key points

The key to the UK policy's success was egalitarianism and consistent, clear, practical nutrition information on radio and in print media. Healthy foods (but not luxuries) were affordable to all. The policy was to ration nothing, however scarce, until there was enough to go round and then to ensure that the ration, however small, was always honoured. Everyone from the woman in a slum to the royal family had ration books and media advice was directed to everyone without targeting a particular social group. It became culturally expected that a pregnant woman should get a larger helping of meat and children would be offered the best bits of the family meal. This influence survived the war. A later study of working class families published in 1963 noted: *". . . these children benefit additionally from the high tea custom, in that they are likely still to be up when father is having his evening meal and to be fed from his plate with titbits of meat or bacon. This extra source of protein foods which seems considerable enough to be mentioned frequently by mothers, is a privilege probably only enjoyed by the youngest child."* [3] This was written in the era of the great protein obsession[4] but is nevertheless sound. Both protein and micronutrients such as iron would be in these 'titbits'.

Appendix IV

ADDITIONAL INFORMATION ON THE SPECIAL SUPPLEMENTAL NUTRITION PROGRAM FOR WOMEN, INFANTS AND CHILDREN (WIC)

The US Congress appropriated US$6.86 billion for WIC in 2009 (cf US$20.6 million in 1974). Costs are met by the federal government, ie the US taxpayer, but individual States negotiate rebates from infant formula manufacturers who bid competitively. The WIC infant formula 'market' is the largest in the world. It is probable that WIC, as much as hospital practices and promotion, has assisted in the decline of breastfeeding.[1] In 2008, 8.2 million people received WIC 'benefits'. In addition to infant formula, WIC provides complementary foods for use before six months which include infant cereals, 'baby food' (ie jars of pureed foods) and juices. Infant cereal is encouraged and promoted in the USA as the principal source of iron in the diet of infants and young children. There is a dilemma that, if these products are withheld from mothers until after six months, infants will be given unsuitable complementary foods. Recent research shows that 70% of infants consume complementary foods before six months despite professional advice.

WIC also provides a package of family foods that reflect the nutritional priorities of the 1950s, ie predominantly high-protein, high-energy foods. In recent years there have been moves to change the WIC food package because it is acknowledged that it has lacked sufficient fresh and diverse fruits and vegetables.[2] The USA now has the highest proportion of overweight people in the world and 30% of adults are obese (cf Japan 2.4%). In the USA, 25.1% of children between 13 and 15 years of age are overweight compared with 7.6% in Holland. Within the USA the prevalence of childhood overweight and obesity is linked to inequality. The more unequal US States will inevitably have more WIC recipients. It is likely that the WIC nutritional programme has contributed to the epidemic of overweight and obesity.[3]

The WIC programme extends to US overseas territories such as American Samoa where overweight, obesity and associated disease are a major public health problem.[4]

REFERENCES

Introduction
1   *The International Code of Marketing of Breast-milk Substitutes* and all subsequent, relevant WHA resolutions (http://www.who.int/nutrition/publications/code_english.pdf), and *The Global Strategy for Infant and Young Child Feeding* (http://www.who.int/nutrition/publications/infantfeeding/9241562218/en/index.html).

Foreword
1   Vidal J. Way out of the woods is into Kenya's trees. *Guardian Weekly,* 5 June, 2009.

Chapter I
1   Sen A. *Poverty and Famines: an essay on entitlement and deprivation.* OUP 1981. Also Kent G (ed). *Global obligations for the right to food.* Rowman & Littlefield, 2008.
2   See: Kent G (ed). *Global obligations for the right to food.* Rowman and Littlefield Publishers, 2008.

Chapter 2
1   Greiner T. *Guidelines for the Marketing of RUSFs for Children.* In Press. Field Exchange. May 2011.
2   Palmer G. *The Politics of Breastfeeding.* Pinter & Martin, 2009.
3   Alipui N. Strong public-private sector partnerships can help reduce undernutrition. www.eldis.org Institute of Development Studies July 2008.
4   Ziegler EE and Fomon SJ. Potential Renal Solute Load of Infant Formulas. *Journal of Nutrition* 1989; 119: 1785-1788.
5   Palmer G. *The Politics of Breastfeeding.* Pinter & Martin, 2009: pp114-116.
6   UN. *The Convention on the Rights of the Child (Article 24 (c)).* 1989.
7   WHO/UNICEF. *The Global Strategy for Infant and Young Child Feeding.* 2003, p18
8   UN. *The Millennium Development Goals.* Report 2007.
9   Cairncross S & Valdmanis V. Water Supply, Sanitation, and Hygiene Promotion. In: *Disease Control Priorities for Developing Countries.* The World Bank Group, 2006: p771-792. Also: Fry K. MSc Dissertation, LSHTM 20008. Also: Personal Communication, Sandy Cairncross, Professor of Environmental Health, LSHTM, 2009.

Chapter 3
1   Alipui N. *Strong public-private sector partnerships can help reduce undernutrition.* www.eldis.org Institute of Development Studies July 2008.
2   See also: Arie S. Hungry for profit. *BMJ* 2010; 341:c5221.
3   Jeffrey Sachs, Jessica Fanzo and Sonia Sachs. Saying "Nuts" to Hunger. www.huffingtonpost.com/jeffrey-sachs/saying-nuts-to-hunger_b_706798.html

Chapter 4
1   Virtual Water. WEM *The Environment Magazine* 14 (6) June 2009.
2   Vidal, John. Fears for the world's poor countries as the rich grab land to grow food. *Guardian,* 4 July 2009.
3   Beddington J. Sustainability and the Perfect Storm. Ninth Annual Lecture Series in Sustainable Development. Cambridge University Department of Engineeering. 2 February 2011.
4   Tolstoy L (1886). Chapter 16 in: *What then must we do.*

Chapter 6
1   Richter J. Public-*Private Partnerships and International health Policy-making.* Ministry of Foreign Affairs of Finland. 2004.
2   See publications of Sarah Blaffer Hrdy: www.hup.harvard.edu.
3   See: Davis M. *Late Victorian Holocausts: El Niño famines and the making of the*

Third World. Verso, 2001 Also: Becker J. *Hungry Ghosts: China's Secret Famine*. John Murray, 1996.

4   The General Assembly of the United Nations. *The Convention on the Rights of the Child*. Adopted 1989.

5   Madeley J. The crisis has a silver lining. *UNICEF News*. 1984.

6   Madeley J. *Food for All*. Zed Books, 2002: pp23-24.

Chapter 7

1   Moynihan P. Dental disease. In *Human Nutrition 11th edition*, eds C Geissler & H Powers, Elsevier, 2005: pp461-478.

2   Sinha R *et al*. Meat intake and mortality, *Arch Intern Med*. 2009;169 (6):562-571.

3   Beardsworth A *et al*. Women, men and food: the significance of gender attitudes and choices. *British Food Journal* 2002; 104 (7): 470-491.

4   Uvnäs Moberg K. *The Oxytocin Factor*. A Merloyd Lawrence Book, Da Capo Press, 2003.

5   UN Protein-Calorie Advisory Group (PAG).

6   McClaren DS. The great protein fiasco. *The Lancet* 1974; 2: 93-6.

7   Aggett P. Harmonising approaches to realigning dietary recommendations. *Maternal & Child Nutrition*. 6: (suppl.2) pp1-2 2010.

8   See: Mann J. Cardiovascular Disease. In Geissler C & Powers H, eds. *Human Nutrition 11th Edition*. Elsevier, 2005.

9   Lutter C. Meeting the challenge to improve complementary feeding. *SCN News* 27 December 2003, pp 4-9.

10 Standing Committee on Nutrition (SCN) 33rd Session (13-17 March, 2006). Tackling the Double Burden of Malnutrition: A Global Agenda. SCN, Geneva, Switzerland.

11 Lawrence Ruth A and Lawrence Robert M. *Breastfeeeding: A Guide for the Medical Profession*. Mosby 5th edition 1999. p 421.

12 Susanna Y *et al*. Timing of solid food introduction and the risk of obesity in pre-school-aged children. *Pediatrics*, Feb 2011. DOI:10.1542/peds.2010-0740.

13 Li R *et al*. Do infants fed from bottles lack self-regulation of milk intake compared with directly breastfed infants? *Pediatrics* 10 May 2010.

14 Prentice AM and Jebb SA. Fast foods, energy density and obesity: a possible mechanistic link. *Obesity Reviews* 14 : (4): 187-194 Nov. 2010.

Chapter 8

1   Lee RB and Daly R, eds. *The Cambridge Encyclopaedia of Hunters and Gatherers*. Cambridge University Press, 2002.

2   Jones M. *Feast: Why Humans Share Food*. Oxford University Press, 2007. See also: Diamond J *Guns, germs and steel*. Vintage, 1997.

Chapter 9

1   Johns T. Dietary diversity, global change, and human health. Proceedings of the symposium "Managing Biodiversity in Agricultural Ecosystems", Montreal, Canada, 8-10 November, 2001.

2   Wilson B. Swindled The dark history of food cheats. John Murray 2008.

3   See Ray Mears website: www.raymears.com

4   Wilkinson R and Pickett K. *The Spirit Level*. Allen Lane, 2009.

5   See Schlosser E. *Fast Food Nation*. Allen Lane and Lawrence F (2008*). Eat your heart out: why the food business is bad for the planet and your health*. Penguin Books, 2001.

Chapter 10

1   Sheiham A. Sweet taste. Paper in progress. Personal Communication June 2011.

Chapter 11

1   *Diet, physical activity and health*. Geneva, World Health Organization, 2002 (documents A55/16 and A55/16 Corr.1). NB: Besides the mortality reduction due to immunisation, there is the protection from disability such as, for example, eye and/ or brain damage from measles: I am in no way suggesting that childhood infections are a good thing, merely a factor to be considered.

2   De Onis M, Garza C, Onyango AW, Borghi E. Journal of Nutrition 2007;137 www.
     who.int/entity/childgrowth/publications/ca_symposium_comparison/en/

Chapter I2

1   Dettwyler KA. A time to wean: the hominid blueprint for the natural age of
     weaning. In: Stuart-Macadam P & Dettwyler KA, eds. *Breastfeeding: Biocultural
     Perspectives.* Aldine de Gruyter, 1995: p.39.
2   Chaparro CM et al. Effect of timing of umbilical cord clamping on iron status in
     Mexican infants: a randomised control trial. *The Lancet* 17 June 2006.
3   Rapley G. Baby-led weaning: a developmental approach to the introduction of
     complementary foods. In Hall Moran V & Dykes F. *Maternal and Infant Nutrition
     and Nurture Controversies and Challenges,* Quay Books, 2006, pp275-298.
4   Wright CM et al. Is baby-led weaning feasible? When do babies first reach out for
     and eat finger foods? *Maternal and Child Nutrition* 7, 2011, pp27-33.
5   Robertson A et al (eds). Food and health in Europe: a new basis for action.
     WHO Regional Publications. European Series. No 96, Copenhagen, 2004. Also:
     Westenhoefer J. Establishing good dietary habits – capturing the minds of children.
     Public Health Nutrition 2000; 4(1A), pp125-129.
6   Jones M. *Feast: Why Humans Share Food.* Oxford University Press, 2007.
7   Turnbull C. *The Mountain People,* 1972. Anthropologist Colin Turnbull describes
     the Ik people of Uganda who left their children to fend for themselves in a harsh
     environment.

Chapter I3

1   Francis Pryor: see publications and websites bbc.co.uk.history.
2   Jelliffe DB et al. The children of the Hadza hunters. *Journal of Pediatrics* 1962;60(6).
3   Ahmed F, Azim A, Akhtaruzzaman M. Vitamin A deficiency in poor, urban,
     lactating women in Bangladesh: factors influencing vitamin A status. *Public Health
     Nutr* 2003; 5,447-52.

Chapter I4

1   Hamosh MS. *Breastfeeding: Unraveling the Mysteries of Mother's Milk* 1999. www.
     Medscape.com/hamosh/w120.hamosh.htm cited in Williams C. The Composition of
     Breastmilk and how it compares with Formula and Cows' milk. *WHO Consultancy
     Review Paper,* 2007 (unpublished).
2   Braun-Fahrländer C. Does the 'hygiene hypothesis' provide an explanation for the
     relatively low prevalence of asthma in Bangladesh? *Int J of Epidem* 2002. 31(2):488-
     489.
3   Food and Agriculture Organization of the United Nations/World Health
     Organization (FAO/WHO) Chapter 13 Iron. In: *Expert consultation on human
     vitamin and mineral requirements.* FAO/WHO 1998.
4   For example: Lorraine Kelly with Anita Bean. *Lorraine Kelly's Baby and Toddler
     Eating Plan.* Virgin Books, 2002.
5   Organix First 'Organic Sweetcorn and Potato' to be given 'from 4 months' and
     endorsed by 'Allergy UK' with 'Free from Gluten' on the label. Purchased 2008.
6   Hamosh MS op cit.
7   Trayhurn P & Stuart Wood I. Diet and genotype interactions – nutritional
     genomics. In *Human Nutrition,* eds. C Geissler & H Powers. Elsevier, 2005, pp537-
     553.
8   Guandolini S. The influence of gluten: weaning recommendations for healthy
     children and children at risk for celiac disease. *Nestlé Nutr Workshop Ser Pediatr
     Program.* 2007;60:139-51. Comment: apologies for using a Nestlé reference but
     this had best information. This author wrote: *"In most developed countries, gluten
     is currently introduced between 4 and 6 months of age, in spite of little evidence
     to support this practice."* Ironic that Nestlé manufactures and promotes gluten-
     containing cereals.
9   Lorri WSM. *Nutritional and microbiological evaluation of fermented cereal weaning*

foods. Department of Food Science, Chalmers University of Technology, Goteborg, Sweden, 1993.

Chapter 15

1   Atkins PJ & Brassley P. Mad cows and Englishmen. *History Today* 1996;46(9):14-7.
2   Hallberg L *et al*. Iron, zinc and other trace elements. In: Garrow JS, James WPT & Ralph A, eds. *Human Nutrition and Dietetics (10th edition)*. Churchill Livingstone 2000: pp177-209.
3   WHO *Management of severe malnutrition: a manual for physicians and other senior health workers*. WHO Geneva, 1999.
4   Reiping EJ. Breast cancer and early contact with bovine milk. Paper presented at Meeting of the *European Society of Gynaecological Oncology*. 1987.
5   Kostraba *et al*. Early exposure to cows' milk and type 1 diabetes mellitus. A critical overview of the clinical literature. *Diabetes Care* 1994;17:13-19.
6   FAO/WHO. *Enterobacter sakazakii* and other microorganisms in powdered infant formula. Meeting Report. Geneva Switzerland, 2-5 February 2004. (FAO/WHO) *Microbiological Risk Assessment Series No. 6*.
7   *BMJ* 2008;337;a1438.
8   IBFAN-ICDC Press Statement. *The Sanlu Fiasco*: 20 September 2008.

Chapter 16

1   Bishop J. Blood, Sweat and Takeaways. BBC 3 26 May 2009. This film made in Kalimantan, Indonesia, depicts conditions in the prawns-for-export industry.
2   Crawford MA *et al*. The role of docosahexaenoic and arachidonic acids as determinants of evolution and hominid brain development. In: Tsukamoto K & Kawamura T *et al*, eds. *Fisheries for Global Welfare and Environment: 5th World Fisheries Congress*. Terrapub Tokyo 2008: pp57–76. See also: Crawford MA. The role of nutrition in human evolution. The Caroline Walker Lecture 2002.
3   Johns T. Dietary diversity, global change, and human health. Proceedings of the symposium "Managing Biodiversity in Agricultural Ecosystems", Montreal, Canada, 8-10 November, 2001.
4   Truswell AS. Diet and nutrition of hunter-gatherers. In *Health and disease in tribal societies*. Ciba Foundation Symposium No.49, Elsevier-Excerpta Medica N. Holland. 1977.
5   Chaparro CM *et al*. Effect of timing of umbilical cord clamping on iron status in Mexican infants: a randomised control trial. *The Lancet* 17 June 2006.
6   Dr Lynn Dicks of the Cambridge Centre for Climate Change and Mitigation Research. *Home Planet*. BBC Radio 4, 7 July 2009.

Chapter 17

1   See Goldacre B. *Bad Science*. Fourth Estate, 2009: pp63-85.
2   McClaren DS. The great protein fiasco. *The Lancet* 1974;2:93-96.
3   Jones M. *Feast: Why Humans Share Food*. Oxford University Press, 2007.
4   Kurlansky C. *Cod: a Biography of the Fish that Changed the World*. Vintage, 1999.
5   Jones M. *Feast: Why Humans Share Food*. Oxford University Press, 2007.

Chapter 18

1   Administrative Order (AO) No. 51: Implementing Rules and Regulations (RIRR) of Executive Order No. 51. Otherwise known as "The Milk Code." 2006-0012 Revised.
2   Sokol E. Implementing national measures. In *The Code Handbook*. ICDC 1997, pp112-133.
3   Kurlansky M. *The Story of Cod*. Vintage, 1999.
4   WHO/UNICEF/ICCIDD Report *Progress Towards the Elimination of Iodine Deficiency Disorders (IDD)*, WHO/NHD/99.4 1999.
5   In Freese L, ed. *Advances in Human Ecology, Vol. 7*. JAI Press Inc. 1998: pp293-312.

Chapter 19

1   Duffield A. Impact of cash relief programme on child caring practices in Meket Wareda, Save the Children UK (unpublished) 2005. Cited in SCF 2007. Running on

empty: poverty and child malnutrition. SCF Briefing.

2   BBC News UK, Living on the Fife Diet, 20 December 2007 and other related websites.

Chapter 20

1   Orr, JB. *Food, health and income: report on a survey of adequacy of diet in relation to income.* Macmillan, 1937. This research led by Sir John Boyd Orr, then Director of the Rowett Research Institute is cited in Le Gros Clark F & Titmuss RM. *Our food problem and its relation to our national defences.* Penguin, 1939. Also cited in Norman J. *Eating for Victory.* Michael O'Mara Books Ltd, 2007.

2   Le Gros Clark F & Titmuss RM. *Our Food Problem and its relation to our national defences.* Penguin Books 1939.

3   Greaves JP. *Food and nutrition policy in Britain during World War II. Turning adversity to advantage.* Internal UNICEF Paper 1984.

Chapter 21

1   Food & Nutrition Service: WIC program: www.fns.usda.gov/wic/

2   Wilkinson R & Pickett K. *The Spirit Level.* Allen Lane, 2009.

3   CIA World Fact Book 2009

4   Devaney B. WIC turns 35: program effectiveness and future directions. Mathematica Policy Research National Invitational Conference of the Early Childhood Research Collaborative Minneapolis, Minnesota. December 7, 2007.

Chapter 22

1   Black RE *et al.* Maternal and child undernutrition 1. Maternal and child undernutrition: global and regional exposures and health consequences. *The Lancet.* 2008; 371:243-260.

2   Hetzel BS. Iodine-deficiency disorders. In: Garrow JS, James WPT & Ralph A. *Human nutrition and dietetics (10ᵗʰ edition).* Churchill Livingstone, 2000: pp621-650.

3   Gogia S & Sachdev HS. Neonatal vitamin A supplementation for prevention of mortality and morbidity in infancy: systematic review of randomised controlled trials. *BMJ* 2009;338:b919.

4   See: Kirkwood B *et al.* Effect of vitamin A supplementation in women of reproductive age on maternal survival in Ghana (ObaapaVitA): a cluster-randomised, placebo-controlled trial. *The Lancet* 2010;375(9726):1640-1649.

5   Gluckman PD & Hanson MA. Living with the past: evolution, development, and patterns of disease. *Science,* 17 September 2004.

6   Quinn V (Director of the Academy for Educational Development (USAID)). Statement made in discussion at *Countdown to 2015 Child Survival Conference.* Senate House, University of London, 13-14 December 2005.

7   Cited in Richter J. *We the people or we the corporations.* IBFAN-GIFA 2003; see also Lhotska L. *Whatever happened to health for all?* IBFAN-GIFA 2008.

8   WHO/UNICEF Strengthening action to improve feeding of infants and young children 6-23 months of age in nutrition and child health programmes. *Report of Proceedings* Geneva, 6-9 October 2008, WHO 2008.

9   Dewey K & Adu-Afarwuah S. Review article: Systematic review of the efficacy and effectiveness of complementary feeding interventions in developing countries. *Maternal and Child Nutrition* 2008, 4:24-85.

10   WHO/UNICEF *The Global Strategy for Infant and Young Child Feeding,* 2003, pp8-9.

Afterword

1   The Alma Ata Declaration may be found on World Health Organisation (WHO) websites.

2   Lhotska L. *Whatever happened to Health for All?* IBFAN-GIFA 2008.

3   Linnecar A. Foreword in Lhotska L. *Whatever happened to Health for All?* GIFA/IBFAN 2008.

Appendix I

1   Davidson A. *The Oxford Companion to Food.* Oxford University Press, 1999.

2   Biologist Dr Lynn Dicks of the Cambridge Centre for Climate Change and Mitigation Research reported these data in BBC Radio 4 'Home Planet'. 7 July 2009. Accessible in Home Planet archives on BBC Radio 4 website.

3   Pharoah P (1984). Endemic Cretinism in the Jimi Valley. Film available on CD Rom from Professor Peter Pharoah, University of Liverpool School of Tropical Medicine, UK.

4   Dr Judith Richter, Personal communication, 2009.

5   DeFoliart G. Insects as Human Food in *Crop Protection* 1992;11: 395-399.

6   Bodenheimer FS. *Insects as Human Food.* The Hague 1951.

7   Davidson A. *The Oxford Companion to Food.* Oxford University Press, 1999.

8   Knell Y. Looking for the next Bill Gates. BBC News Channel, 10 July 2009.

Appendix II

1   Sharp P. Minerals and trace elements. In: *Human Nutrition.* C Geissler & H Powers, eds. Elsevier, 2005: pp231-250.

2   Hartmann P. Winthrop Professor of Biochemistry & Molecular Biology, University of Western Australia. Personal communication, 2000.

3   Chaparro CM *et al.* Effect of timing of umbilical cord clamping on iron status in Mexican infants: a randomised control trial. *The Lancet* 2006;367: 1997-2004.

4   Dunn P. Clamping the umbilical cord. *AIMS Journal* 2004/5; 16(4): 8-9.

5   Beardsworth A *et al.* Women, men and food: the significance of gender for nutritional attitudes and choices. *British Food Journal* 2002; 104 (7):470-91.

6   Hallberg L et al. Iron, zinc and other trace elements. In Garrow JS, James WPT & Ralph A, eds. *Human Nutrition and Dietetics.* Churchill Livingstone, 2000: pp177-209.

Appendix III

1   'Supersizers go to World War Two', BBC 2 TV,2008.

2   Veal I. *Recipes of the 1940s* cited in Norman J. 1943.
Other sources of these statements are: Longmate N. *How we lived then: a history of everyday life during the Second World War.* Arrow Books, 1971. Norman J. *Eating for Victory: reproductions of official Second World War instruction leaflets.* Michael O'Mara Books Ltd, 2007. Kurlansky M. *Cod: a biography of the fish that changed the world.* Vintage, 1999. Greaves JP. Food and Nutrition policy in Britain during World War II. Turning adversity to advantage. UNICEF Internal Document 1984.

3   Newson J and Newson E. *Infant care in an urban community.* George Allen and Unwin, 1963.

4   MClaren DS. The great protein fiasco. *The Lancet* 1974;2:93-6.

Appendix IV

1   Kent G. WIC's promotion of infant formula in the United States. *International Breastfeeding Journal* 2006; 198:1-14.

2   www.fns.usda.gov/fns

3   US National Survey of Children's Health cited in Wilkinson R & Pickett K. *The Spirit Level.* Allen Lane, 2009.

4   Lang S. Report on Mother and Child Health in American Samoa. WHO 2003.

INDEX

introduced in wartime UK 82
and long-term food insecurity 73
marketing situation 15–16, 61*, 74, 93
some complementary foods really *de
facto* breastmilk substitutes 25, 49, 56
British food rationing 81–2, 89, 90,
110–12
brucellosis 60*

canned fish 41
carbohydrate foods 32
cardiovascular disease 33, 51
cash crops 28, 63
cashew nuts, processing 41
cassava (manioc)
containing goitrogens 40*
and cyanide content 76
low in protein 33*
poisonous unless processed 75
pros and cons as staple 43
caterpillars, eating 99, 101
cats, eating 66
cereals
appropriateness for babies 54–9
'cerealisation' 67
fortification of 55, 56–7, 58
low in key nutrients 55–6
not ideal first foods 55–6
phytates 57–9, 108
removal of husk 57–8
as staple foods 17, 33*, 55–7, 66
'whiteness', preference for 58, 66
wholegrain 57–8
Challen, Dr Robert 75*
cheese 32, 60, 64, 75
chewing, necessary for introducing
complementary foods 49
child development and readiness for
complementary foods 49–50
children
consumption of meat/ animal foods 31,
68
not getting the best food 13
priority for best foods 82, 112
China
insect consumption 64, 99
and marketing of industrialised foods
66–7
milk scandal 61
Christian Aid 21*
cochineal 101
cocoa beans, processing 41
cod, 'who ate the cod?' 22
Codes of Marketing of Breastmilk
Substitutes 74
coeliac disease 58
complementary feeding
accustomisation 24
definition of in this book 9*
definitions in local laws 74
general description of 24–6
marketing situation the same as for

breastmilk substitutes 93
need for initiative and energy from
mother/ caregiver 87
need for water supply 16
and relationship to mothers' nutrition
87
contamination
branding aims to protect consumers 41
China Sanlu case (melamine in milk)
61
food hygiene 9*, 17–19, 25, 87
reduced risk in RUTFs 16
and seafood 63
of water sources 28
Convention on the Rights of the Child
(CRC) 18, 28
cord-cutting, delayed 48, 50, 64, 106–7
cows' milk *see* animal milks
Crawford, Michael 63
Cuba, child health improvements in 89
cultural attitudes
affecting how children are fed 14, 24,
65–8
eating molluscs/ insects 64, 99, 100–1

dairy industry
protection of 61
and safety of methods 61–2
Danone 90
Davidson, Dr Alan 99, 100
delayed umbilical cord cutting 48, 50, 64,
106–7
dental caries 31, 81
'developing' countries
statistics 23
use of term 'developing world' 89–90
developmental reflexes in children 49
diabetes (type 1)
and early contact with cows' milk 61
and early introduction of gluten-
containing cereals 58
and energy-dense foods 87
disease-protection
breastfeeding for 25
childhood illness and obesity 46
different diets protect against different
diseases 33
food hygiene 9*, 17–19, 25, 87
nomadic lifestyle 51
diseases of affluence 31
distribution of food/ equality *see* food
distribution
diverse diet, humans evolved to thrive on
32–3, 40, 50, 52, 64
Don't let Dad get all the meat 81, 107
drinking water, essential 16
dynamic food systems 42

early cord clamping 48, 50, 64, 106–7
early introduction of complementary
foods 86–7, 113
eating disorders 25

economics *see also* food industry
  farmland in poor countries producing
    food for rich 22, 28
  of nutrition programmes 90
  people better fed in economic
    downturns 28 *see also* wartime UK
    rationing
  profit motives 41, 88
  of RUTFs 21, 23
education, as key to better diet 29, 44, 79
energy density, (erroneous) focus on 33
energy needs of small children 33
energy-dense/nutrient-poor foods 25, 33,
  34, 35, 87
enrichment of foods *see* fortification of
  foods
entitlements
  to food 13–14, 79
  to water 15–19
enzymes
  amylase (enzyme) 57
  lactase 60
Ethiopia 41*, 57, 79
evidence-based public health 56, 82
evolution 33, 40–4, 52, 57, 60, 63
exporting food
  countries with undernutrition exporting
    to rich 22, 28
  Irish grain 13
  Irish seafood 67
  prawns 63
extended breastfeeding (beyond 2 years)
  16, 25, 48–9

factory-made foods *see* processed foods
fair distribution of food/ equality *see* food
  distribution
family foods, young children enjoying
  50, 82
famine *see also* RUTFs (Ready-to-Use-
  Therapeutic-Foods)
  common occurrence in human history
    27
  famine foods, cassava as 43
  famine foods, danger of 'branding'
    foods as 101
Fanzo, Jessica 21
FAO/WHO guidelines 55
farming *see also* agriculture
farming/ agriculture
  cash crops 28, 63
  environmental effects 22
  farmland in poor countries producing
    food for rich 22, 28
  history of 39
  monocultures 42
fast food 35, 44, 77
fat storage 46–7
fats 32
fatty acids 63
fatty foods 45
favism 32*

fermentation
  enhances nutrition of food 59, 75, 109
  often (wrongly) considered unhygienic
    27, 59*
fibre
  as iron inhibitor 108
  not needed by infants 57
Fife Diet 79–80
Fildes, Valerie 48*
first foods
  cereals not good as 17, 54–9
  molluscs, insects and small animals
    ideal 52, 57
  purees/ 'baby food' not necessary 33,
    50, 54
flesh foods
  as best form of iron 55, 107
  biologically most appropriate first foods
    57
  saltiness 45
  typically not given to children 55–6
folk memories 67
food aid 21 *see also* RUTFs (Ready-
  to-Use-Therapeutic-Foods); WIC
  (US Special Supplemental Nutrition
  Program for Women, Infants and
  Children)
food distribution
  within families 13, 24, 31, 81–2, 107, 112
  globally 22–3, 24, 67–8
  government controlled 81–2, 83–4, 85
  rationing in UK wartime 81–2
food hygiene 9*, 17–19, 25, 87
food industry
  baby food companies 74, 90, 93–4
  Danone 90
  deskilling families transfers power to
    big business 90
  Gerber 74
  Nestlé 66, 90*
  politics of food industry 27–9
  transnational food companies 41, 93–4
'food literacy' 22
food security
  breastfeeding a form of 48
  improved by wartime rationing 81–2,
    110
  long-term food insecurity 73, 88
  trade-off with good nutrition 42
  and undernutrition 20, 28–9
food sharing (families) 21, 24, 31–2, 50
food storage
  fermented foods 59
  and nutrient content 74–5
  vitamins potentially better in frozen/
    stored food than 'fresh' 74–5
food-survival skills, lacking 42–3
foraging/ wild foods 8, 39, 45, 76, 110
formula *see* artificial milks (formula milk)
Formula 100 (F100) 15*
fortification of foods
  cereals 55, 56–7, 58

ABOUT **PINTER & MARTIN**

Pinter & Martin is an independent book publisher based in London, with distribution throughout the world. We specialise in psychology, pregnancy, birth and parenting, fiction and yoga, and publish authors who challenge the status quo, such as Elliot Aronson, Grantly Dick-Read, Ina May Gaskin, Stanley Milgram, Guillermo O'Joyce, Michel Odent, Gabrielle Palmer, Stuart Sutherland and Frank Zappa.

For more information, visit www.pinterandmartin.com

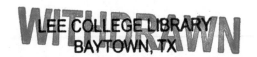